NOT TRYING

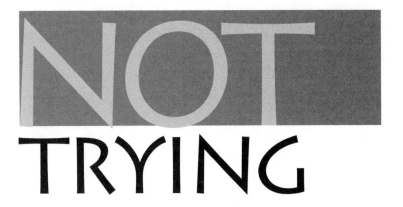

NOT TRYING

INFERTILITY, CHILDLESSNESS, AND AMBIVALENCE

KRISTIN J. WILSON

VANDERBILT UNIVERSITY PRESS

Nashville

© 2014 by Vanderbilt University Press
Nashville, Tennessee 37235
All rights reserved
First printing 2014

This book is printed on acid-free paper.
Manufactured in the United States of America

Book and cover design by Rich Hendel
Composition by E.T. Lowe, Nashville, TN

Library of Congress Cataloging-in-Publication Data on file
LC control number   2014007695
LC classification number   HQ755.8.W544 2014
Dewey class number   306.87—dc23
ISBN 978-0-8265-1996-2 (cloth)
ISBN 978-0-8265-1997-9 (paperback)
ISBN 978-0-8265-1998-6 (ebook)

CONTENTS

ACKNOWLEDGMENTS

My name is on this book and any errors inside are my own. But many people helped me complete it. If it were a movie, the credits would roll on and on. I first have to thank the women willing to take the time to share their thoughts and feelings with me. Without them there would be no book. My mentor and dear friend, Wendy Simonds, guided and supported me from beginning to end. I extend deep appreciation to my editor, Michael Ames, for his thoughtful feedback and patient tutelage. Thank you very much to the anonymous reviewers, to Ralph LaRossa, and to Elisabeth Burgess for their comments, which helped me improve the manuscript. My home institutions, Cabrillo College and Georgia State University, provided material support. Seline Szkupinski-Quiroga, another scholar working on this topic, kindly provided some key early advice about participant recruitment. Scholars from the History of Consciousness Department at the University of California–Santa Cruz welcomed me into their writing group and read some of the chapters, providing useful insights.

At the beginning of this project, I was fully immersed in fertility treatment. My then partner and I eventually gave up and pursued adoption. After a year-long training and home-study period, we took home a baby boy through the California fost-adopt program. Thirteen months later, his birth mother relinquished another newborn, our son's brother. Evan and Leo are now six and five, respectively, and I have been working on this book their entire lives. This was made possible by the nurturing childcare provided by Adriana Castillo and the staff of Casa de

Aprendizaje, by Ashley George of Honalee Children's Center, and by Lupe Cortes, Heather Elrick-Forbes, and all the staff at Cabrillo Children's Center.

Many friends, family, and colleagues provided emotional support, but I especially want to thank Mary Arterburn, Anthony Garcia, Paul Conte, Meredith Marine, Allison Gonzalez, Rebecca Green, Meadow Gibbons, Karinn Pearson, Melissa Workman, Jackie Logg, Raneta Pomroy, Chuck Smith, the "Cruzmoms," and Mom and Dad.

NOT TRYING

ENTERING OTHERHOOD

"How're you doing with your plight?" asked my new fertility doctor when he entered the exam room. While sitting fully clothed awaiting this initial consultation, I looked over the thick files that constituted my fertility history up to that point (it would get much thicker in the coming years). There was much more to the experience than these papers indicated. The files included the results of the examination by an OB/GYN, who palpated my reproductive organs and performed tests for HIV, gonorrhea, and chlamydia, all State of Georgia requirements to receive intrauterine insemination (IUI)—tests not required, of course, for conventional attempts at pregnancy.

There were files from the dozen or so IUIs I underwent at a for-profit clinic, a place I eventually left as it became clear that the timing of my cycles invariably failed to match the schedule of the moonlighting doctor. (The procedure is quick and simple: insert sperm-filled syringe into the cervical os and push the plunger. Yet it is a felony in Georgia to perform it oneself—or for a friend or partner to do so.)

Several pages documented the extensive blood work and medication regimen accompanying the next three cycles that took place at a nonprofit, women-centered, more technologically outfitted clinic. Ultrasound printouts of multiple, robust, fertility-drug-enhanced egg follicles—one cycle produced nine primed eggs—and records describing the healthy, motile, "normal" donor sperm were attached to brief, scrawled notations attesting to the negative results. The medical staff omitted any mention of the 105 degree fever that spiked half an hour after the last insemination, nor did they record the prescription for emergency high-dosage antibiotics used to kill the apparent infection. I would have to relay this dramatic incident to the new doctor myself.

My records did not include the semen tests, blood work, and surgical procedures that my partner went through. His diagnosis of irreversible sterility mentioned on all my medical forms was upsetting enough, but the subsequent discovery (pre-Obamacare) that we could no longer purchase private health insurance for him as a result was both appalling and absurd. Nowhere among the medical memos could one find any data about my or my partner's feelings of inadequacy, the disruption of our expected life plan, and the destabilization of our gendered expectations of biological and genetic motherhood and fatherhood. Also missing from the files was my frustration at the paradoxical loss of control over my body at the same time obedient hypercontrol was prescribed. To wit, the daily pattern involved taking my basal body temperature; noting every abdominal twinge; ingesting chaste tree oil, dandelion tinctures, milk thistle caplets, and Clomid tablets (an ovulation drug); inserting progesterone suppositories; and suffering concomitant hot flashes, night sweats, irritability, and—worst of all—dry mouth. On a monthly basis, we dropped everything to race to the clinic when the urine dipstick yielded a "high fertility" readout on my Clearblue-brand ovulation computer. The clinics listed only the dosages for Clomid and progesterone. One could not discern from these documents the cyclical buildup of hope, followed by tearful disappointment and then hope built anew.

Despite all the emotional, financial, and medical trials experienced over the previous several years of infertility, the doctor's question bothered me. His choice of the word *plight* implied victimhood, a label I rejected. Still, his inquiry suggested that he empathized with me, that he was not going to dismiss the psycho-emotional and social impact of infertility. His purpose in asking the question may have been to assess my emotional state or to solicit a summary of the relevant tests, treatments, and procedures that I already had completed or tried. I responded, "I don't really think of it as a plight."

"Well, journey, then," he replied as he barely suppressed an eye roll and exhaled with exaggerated patience. Although the advice literature suggests to infertile women that they approach treatment as a journey to self-discovery and to well-earned, meant-to-be motherhood, this concept also failed to capture my experience. The daily hassles and discomforts; the monthly highs and lows; the frustrating, painful, time-consuming en-counters with harried doctors, bored clinicians, and intrusive medical protocols—all felt less like a journey and more like a slog. The opposing concepts of plight and journey evoke re-spective images of an unwitting victim who lacks agency or an adventuresome traveler uninhibited by institutions and social structures.

Constructing the Infertile Woman

Some describe infertility as a "yuppie disease." Women who seek fertility treatment in the United States do tend to fit a narrow demographic. Like me, they are usually white, middle class, well educated, and married. They appear to fit into a socially con-structed paradigm of what may be called the "Infertile Woman," a career-oriented woman who delayed childbearing and, now overwrought and desperate for motherhood, is able to tap into the social, cultural, and financial capital needed to make use of medically assisted conception or, perhaps, to eventually pursue adoption. For its part, the treatment industry cultivates a more positive image of a savvy consumer capable of selecting from an array of ever more elaborate fertility technologies and alternative cures like acupuncture.

Scholars, support groups, and caregivers alike portray suffering as a universal experience for infertile women. Harvard University business professor Deborah Spar writes in *The Baby Business*, "Regardless of the cause, however, and regardless of age, infertility wreaks inestimable havoc on those who suffer from it" (2006, 16). INCIID, the InterNational Council on Infertility Information Dissemination, is a well-known information clearinghouse and gateway to fertility clinics. The top of their webpage contains a picture of a smiling woman alongside the quotation, "INCIID [pronounced "inside"] is the one place where I can go and feel understood when dealing with the most painful part of my life—infertility" (*INCIID*). Their logo, incidentally, contains a line drawing of a man and woman in business attire holding hands. This image suggests that their target audience consists of professional married couples—that is, yuppies. *Fertility and Sterility* and *Human Reproduction*, the primary medical journals on infertility, regularly publish articles on the psychological consequences of infertility, devoting subcategories to "psychology and counseling," services often required by clinics providing fertility treatment. These articles typically make the case that infertility is a major life disruption, and they examine fertility distress from many angles. Advertisements in these same journals tap into images of the desperate and hopeful Infertile Woman. For example, a common ad for fertility medications depicts a white-coated, bespectacled, and fatherly doctor holding a chart and addressing a well-to-do, worried-looking young couple seated in his office. The caption reads, "You are their only hope."

Conceive Magazine, a bimonthly consumer publication and

website, contains many articles like the one that reads, "The very diagnosis of infertility brings with it a sense of grief and loss" (Lombardo 2009: 30). A back-cover ad for the pharmaceutical company Serono depicts a married woman's left hand on her torso with the wistful caption, "I wish my pants didn't fit. I wish I were tired. I wish I were pregnant." The medical practice Georgia Reproductive Specialists provides this advice to its patients and its patients' friends: "Remember that a fertility issue is a *crisis* [emphasis in original]" (*www.ivf.com*, March 2013).

Social research also paints a grim picture of the infertility experience. As with my own anxious experience with infertility, treatment seekers often feel unhappy and disempowered (Becker 2000; Franklin 1997; Harwood 2007; Haynes and Miller 2003). In her review and (brilliant) philosophical treatise on the topic, Charis Thompson (2005, 55) notes, "involuntary childlessness is recognized as being one of the greatest forms of unhappiness and loss an adult woman might have to endure." Indeed, a random sample of 580 midwestern women demonstrates a negative association between lifetime infertility and life satisfaction (McQuillan et al. 2011). Among infertile and childless couples, women usually report more emotional pain than do men (Abbey et al. 1992; Greil 1991). The content summaries on the back covers of two newer edited volumes on infertility begin with these statements: "Worldwide, over 75 million people are involuntarily childless, a devastating experience for many with significant consequences for the social and psychological well-being of women in particular" (Culley et al. 2009) and "Reproductive disruptions, like infertility, pregnancy loss, adoption, and childhood disability, are among the most distressing experiences in people's lives" (Inhorn, ed., 2009). Between the covers these authors and editors, who are established leaders in the field, proffer rich analyses based on thorough and well-funded research—in fact, funded sometimes by the manufacturers of infertility medications. But the books advertise, at least, an emphasis on "distress" and "devastation."

Deconstructing the Infertile Woman

Infertility is a life crisis. Childlessness is either a tragedy or a (dubious) chosen lifestyle, in which case it may be called being "childfree." Women are meant to be mothers.

These truisms fall apart when talking to real women outside the treatment context.

After all, only 36 percent of infertile women seek advanced treatment (CDC 2004). The lived experience of infertile and/or involuntarily childless poor women, women of color, gay and queer women, and single women—in short, those largely excluded from an entrenched societal proscription against childlessness, or what Nancy Felipe Russo (1976) calls the "motherhood mandate"—provides a fresh perspective.

What is understood in sociology and anthropology about infertile women and couples generally comes from a fairly homogenous pool that funnels in members who have an interest in medically assisted procreation. It is crucial to point out that most ethnographic studies of infertility and involuntary childlessness in the context of procreative technology share a certain recruitment etiology (Abbey et al. 1992; Franklin 1997; Becker 2000; Letherby 2002a; Greil 1991; Lasker and Borg 1994; Sandelowski 1991; Szkupinski-Quiroga 2002, 2007; Harwood 2007). Respondents come from two primary sources: fertility clinics (in the United Kingdom and United States) and the RESOLVE organization, a national support group and information clearinghouse that originated in Boston in 1974. RESOLVE, criticized by informants as exclusionary in one of these studies (Szkupinski-Quiroga 2002), simultaneously contributes to the medicalization and psychologization (van

Balen 2002) of childlessness. Fertility clinics may foster the same effect.

For this book I interviewed twenty-five women who belong to socially marginalized groups, who are not seeking treatment, and who see themselves as "off course" in terms of the social expectation that they should become or should have become mothers. Their diverse experiences differ from that of fertility strugglers and their attitudes offer a perhaps more liberating way of thinking about infertility and childlessness.

Finding the Infertile Woman

Women who are infertile do not look different from anyone else. Since I wanted to talk to women from a range of social backgrounds who are also among the infertile majority who do not seek treatment, I had to find them by meeting them personally or by word of mouth. The primary challenge of recruitment was the word—indeed the concept of—*infertility* itself. Everyone knew what it was, but only a few of the respondents truly identified as such. I tried asking around for women who "wanted kids but couldn't have them." After conducting a few hard-won interviews, it began to dawn on me that women were so ambivalent about whether they wanted children or not, so disinvested with medicalization and its terminology, and so pragmatic and unwilling to name their current fertility status that the concept simply did not resonate with them. To them "infertility" was something that others—namely IVF seekers—experienced even while these respondents also rejected the idea that they had chosen childlessness.

I was seeking a hidden population. Partly to avoid the stigma, the women would not say exactly that they were infertile or involuntarily childless. It was typical for me to receive a phone call from a potential respondent who, when asked whether she was infertile, would almost invariably say something to this effect:

"Well, I'm not *really* infertile; not for sure." If there were no "infertile" women from marginalized groups identifying themselves, then I had to expand that criterion. I began also looking for women who did not have children. By choosing not to specify whether or not the childlessness was voluntary or involuntary, I figured, I could find more participants. This stratagem worked. I discovered that "voluntary" childlessness meant almost as little to the women I spoke with as "involuntary" childlessness and "infertility" did. The Appendix provides a demographic summary of the study participants.

The women who agreed to be interviewed chose the location of the interviews, often their own homes. That comfortable setting fostered intimate disclosures. Most of the time, we sat on the floor or on couches, often drinking tea and being moved to tears.

Few of the women I talked with had any questions for me, but one asked, "Do *you* want kids?" All along, I had been probing for her thoughts on motherhood and her perceptions of why people have children. Self-satisfied, she exclaimed "I *knew* it!" upon hearing my affirmative answer. She showed me the pronatalist bias inherent in my line of questioning. In a similar vein, psychologist Maggíe Kirkman (2001, 523) reported that the infertile Australian women she interviewed chafed at the suggestion that they should "justify their desire to become mothers." Although I was not requiring women to justify their situations, my questions did spark a bit of surprise and a great deal of introspection as women considered their infertility and childlessness in new ways. Several of them emphasized that they have chosen not to think about or dwell on that status, and for a few of the older women, it seemed they were thinking and talking about it for the first time. Almost all of them thanked me for what a couple of them dubbed "free therapy."

Throughout my time in the field, I was undergoing fertility treatment and struggling with depression over my childlessness. I took note of how the other women coped and how they processed similar experiences. They offered multiple streams of wisdom, born of quite different life stories and pathways to infertility or childlessness. Not only did they help shed light on the research questions, but their perspectives were also unexpectedly therapeutic for *me*.

Reconceiving Infertility and Involuntary Childlessness

"Infertility" and "childlessness" are overlapping, loaded terms that connote an array of social meanings about motherhood and women's roles. To start with, the standard medical definition of infertility is hardly an objective, scientific one; it is through and through a social and cultural construction (Greil et al, "Social Construction," 2011). In medical usage it means that a woman has not gotten pregnant after six months of "unprotected" and "regular" heterosexual sex if she is under thirty-five years of age, or after twelve months if thirty-five or older. This inexact rule of thumb assumes failure to conceive to be the result of mechanical, hormonal, or other physiological problems and does not always account for frequency of sex, timing, time elapsed since taking oral or injectable contraceptives, multiple partners and their fertility, or sexual behavior patterns like position, withdrawal, and washing. In addition, a scan of cross-cultural experiences with infertility indicates that in some societies a woman may experience infertility if she does not give birth to a son, if she does not bear a child free from perceived defects, or if she does not conceive in a matter of months following marriage (Greil 1991; van Balen and Inhorn 2002).

Disease etiology in infertility is notoriously difficult to trace, with about 20 percent of cases designated as "unexplained." Moreover, the accepted delineation of infertility does not distinguish between those who wish to get pregnant and those who do not. In actuality, one woman's infertility may be another's good fortune. Not all who seek medically assisted conception (either low-tech procedures and drugs or advanced reproductive technologies) are technically infertile. They may simply lack a fertile male partner: they may be single women, lesbians, celibates, or the otherwise fertile half of a heterosexual couple. The National Survey for Family Growth (NFSG) survey by the Centers for Disease Control (CDC), which lists infertility figures only for married women aged fifteen to forty-four years (defined as the childbearing years), puts forward the broader notion of "impaired fecundity," a concept that includes married and unmarried women who report problems getting pregnant and problems sustaining pregnancy. According to the latest available NSFG (2006–2010) figures, 11.9 percent (7.4 million) of all American women aged fifteen to forty-four experienced "impaired fecundity," and 6 percent of *married* American women were diagnosed as "infertile." Infertile diagnoses are down from 7.4 percent in NSFG statistics gathered in 2002. About 14 percent of childless married American women reported that they were infertile. Based on European population surveys (e.g., Boivin et al. 2007), 15–20 percent is an oft-used—but debated—estimate for current levels of medically diagnosed infertility (Greil 2009; Guzick and Swan 2006; Stephen and Chandra 2006). An international survey estimates that 9 percent of individuals worldwide are infertile (Boivin et al. 2007). Despite breathless reports to the contrary (e.g., Gregory 2007; Spar 2006)—there are distinct moralizing and financial interests in exaggerating the problem—the rates of infertility appear to be fairly consistent over time and across societies, although poverty, racism, and uneven access to quality health care lead to much higher rates of infertility among certain marginalized groups (Inhorn, ed., 2009; Nsiah-Jefferson and Hall 1989).

Drawing conclusions from the published numbers is tricky because infertility is itself a slippery concept, a hazy diagnosis.

Its operationalization is problematic. There is a world of difference, for instance, between polycystic ovarian syndrome (PCOS) or a malformed uterus caused by in utero exposure to the drug DES (two well-known reasons for female-factor infertility), and, say, easily remedied subfertility resulting from the male partner's sperm-reducing affinity for jockey shorts, laptops, or hot tubs. Whether infertility can be "cured" or not is also unclear. Hysterosalpingograms (HSGs)—a (sometimes painful) process of shooting dye into the fallopian tubes to test their openness—may unblock tubes for some, consequently restoring fertility via a happy side-effect of a diagnostic tool. Clomiphene citrate (also known as Clomid) stimulates many a reluctant ovary to produce viable eggs—and occasionally causes a lethal overproduction of eggs. (Treatments can introduce greater harm than help at times). In vitro fertilization bypasses the tubes and requires only a functioning uterus. The proper hormone balance is approximated pharmaceutically. All manner of surgeries, procedures, and drugs exist to enhance a woman's chances of becoming pregnant. A woman can be fertile at one age, infertile later on, and then fertile yet again—with medical intervention and sometimes without it—before eventually aging out of fertility. Infertility is not stable as a medical or analytical category; therefore, it should not be surprising that neither does it confer a static identity. My respondents' stories cast doubt on the common assumption (and self-fulfilling prophecy) of infertility as a default identity and an inevitably devastating experience.

Medically assisted fertilization and adoption are two ways for infertile women to become mothers. These options do not cure; rather, they alleviate the social condition of *involuntary childlessness*. This term is popular with feminist researchers and other social scientists for several reasons: (1) it is a substitute for "infertility" that recognizes the condition as a social one, not intrinsically biological or medical; (2) it includes a wider spectrum of women (i.e., singles and lesbians who do not have procreative sex with biological males); (3) it obscures the "blame" for the condition (its origin as "female-factor" or "male-factor" is less relevant to women's experience of the condition); and (4) it is thought to be less stigma laden. Women are thought to suffer from involuntary childlessness or else be *voluntarily childless*. Another option, the imperfect adjective *childfree*, which sounds like there are no children at all in one's life, at least confers some agency to women with the condition.

For all the clinical-sounding vocabulary surrounding the word nowadays, *infertile* is inescapably associated with barrenness, emptiness, unproductiveness, a lack. Its linguistic opposite, *fertile*, means bountiful, rich, abundant, lush, prolific, and luxuriant. The former designation can be a powerful stigma, signifying loss and inadequacy, whereas the latter confirms one's rightful place in the generative circle of life: as a mother, a nurturer, and giver of life. Similarly, *pregnant* means full. Logically, not pregnant is empty; infertile women are thought to be unfulfilled. Motherhood, in this discourse, signifies the ultimate in fulfillment. Indeed, the Standard North American Family (Smith 1993), that most basic family form—as socially constructed and glorified—consists of a provider-father, a devoted mother, and their offspring. The woman in this family represents the ideal for all women.

Significantly, involuntary childlessness is not necessarily final, and it does not necessarily result from infertility. It is inappropriate to label celibates, singles, and lesbians as "infertile" when the functioning potential of their reproductive systems is unknown. Extending this logic, male-factor infertility (or a boyfriend's or husband's refusal to have children) does not always doom the woman partner to "courtesy infertility" or involuntary childlessness: she can switch partners and some women do just that. And, as I imply above, women's fertility status can change unpredictably, without obvious medical reasons.

The poles of voluntary and involuntary childlessness are just as arbitrary as fertile and infertile. *Voluntary* suggests that a woman makes a conscious choice to forgo motherhood, to give up having children, perhaps, the story goes, in favor of career ambitions or other supposed self-indulgences. Hidden are the myriad and many nonchoices that lead to that presumed decision. For example, is childlessness *voluntary* when a woman never finds the right partner, when she dislikes sex but would otherwise like to have children, or when she lacks the financial position or social support to raise children as she thinks one should? Is childlessness still *involuntary* if a woman refuses to use assisted reproductive technologies (ARTs) that are available to her or when she changes her mind after having her tubes tied? What of the intent of women who *do* have children? Researchers and the general public often fail to consider whether motherhood is voluntary or involuntary for the simple fact that we fall into thinking that it is the natural order of things. Childlessness is the deviant status. At least that is the case for women. In contemporary American society, women are thought to fall into one of three camps: (1) mothers (along a spectrum of bad and good mothers); (2) the desperate and damaged infertile (curable through amazing technological miracles or, less desirably, via heartwarming adoptions); or (3) the militantly childfree (often suspected of careerism and/or lesbianism). The reality, of course, is much more complex.

Whether a woman is called infertile, involuntarily or voluntarily childless, a nonmother, or childfree, the available labels refer to something that is missing. She is *not* fertile or *not* the mother of a child. She is less that child or free from children. In either case, others see her as a woman who disrupts her prescribed role, who does not fit, who must be repaired, pitied, or, at least, explained.

Addressing Infertility and Involuntary Childlessness

Infertility is big business. The industry in the United States generates billions of dollars annually (Spar 2006). Market analysts (e.g., Buscom.com, Marketdata Enterprises, Inc., Medtech Insight) report that infertility was a four-billion-dollar industry in 2010 with growth projections between 10 and 36 percent annually. The global market for just the infertility drugs and devices (not including services) is projected to reach $4.8 billion in the next few years (by 2017) (Letourneau 2012). As of 2006, 483 fertility clinics in the United States provided assisted reproductive technology (ART), with IVF topping the list of services. The number of private physicians and small clinics that provide relatively low-tech treatment, like the IUI procedures I tried, number in the thousands (Spar 2006). The large number of articles published monthly in the American Society of Reproductive Medicine's (ASRM) flagship journal *Fertility and Sterility* attest to the fact that new technologies, pharmaceuticals, and tests are constantly being developed to treat infertility. There is also a booming cottage industry in the publication of self-help, complementary medicine, and advice books. At the vanguard are refined egg-freezing techniques and preimplantation genetic diagnosis (PGD) that laboratory experts can use to ensure that the largest, prescreened ova—perhaps even donated by a (financially compensated) twenty-something Ivy League graduate—are individually fertilized by intracytoplasmic sperm injection (ICSI) with similarly prescreened sperm, possibly attained surgically from a subfertile male partner via testicular sperm extraction (TESE). Next, the resulting in vitro–produced embryos are selected for genetic quality—Steinberg (1997) notes the "eugenic logic of IVF"—and then placed in the consumer-patient's uterus. Deborah Spar (2006) likens the industry to that of luxury goods. Only fifteen states mandate insurance coverage for infertility, possibly with the complicity of fertility clinics which enjoy the fiscal fruits of low supply and high demand. Most women who want the services have to pay exorbitant sums out of pocket. A single cycle of the PGD protocol mentioned above would cost upwards of forty thousand dollars in most cases.

Within this growing industry sector is a burgeoning subspecialty in reproductive tourism. In contrast to the United Kingdom and Australia, where many of the tourist-patients originate, there is remarkably little government regulation in the infertility industry in the United States. America's particular history created the circumstances wherein reproductive politics constitute proverbial hot potatoes for lawmakers. On the one hand, they have to consider the many well-to-do, well-connected (mostly white) constituents who rely on ART for family building, the enriched and empowered medical specialists who serve these patients, and the groundswell of public and scientific support for stem cell research, which has an ancillary and logical connection to ART. On the other hand, legislators and other elected officeholders must contend with perennial agitation from antichoice religious conservatives who are already in paroxysms over the hundreds of thousands of stem cells and frozen embryos that continue to proliferate (Mundy 2007). Avoidance is the prudent and prevailing strategy. Some see it as a Wild West industry that continues to grow rapidly in ways that are largely unchecked. Doctors at California clinics, for instance, were accused of stealing unclaimed frozen eggs and giving them to patients who could not produce their own (Dodge and Geis 2003). Opportunities abound for both abuse (like charlatanism and dangerous experimentation) and for emancipatory use (like lesbian and queer family building) of these technologies.

Foster care and adoption have been conceptualized as non-medical alternatives to infertility or involuntary childlessness (Altstein and Simon 2001; Traver 2008). It is important to note, though, that many adopters first attempt to get pregnant with medical assistance, often exhausting their medical options and nearly emptying their bank accounts by paying for several cycles of IVF (Jacobson 2008). Adoption occupies the bottom tier in the hierarchy of routes to parenthood: it is frequently the last resort, and there are numerous barriers to access and to success (Fisher 2003).

Like medical infertility treatment, adoption is a growing business in which demand exceeds supply. There is a dearth of healthy, white babies, the preferred children for the white, middle-class couples who make up 90 percent of the population of prospective adoptive parents. Roughly 60 percent of the available domestic children are black, Latino, or classified as racially mixed. To encourage foster care and adoption of these and other "special needs" children (who also include children with medical or mental health conditions, sibling groups, and youngsters over age two), the federal government and most states provide financial incentives such as tax credits, free health insurance for the children, and monthly stipends. But most adopters want healthy infants (Rothman 2000b). These prospective parents also wish to avoid the "risk" associated with adopting children from birth mothers who may change their minds or who may demand more of a relationship than the adoptive parents want to accommodate (Dorow 2006; Rothman 2000b; Jacobson 2008).

International adoption—peaking in the early 2000s—enables a supply stream of twenty thousand babies who come to the United States each year with no birth-family strings attached (Bureau of Consular Affairs 2008). Domestic adoptions number about one hundred thousand children. Half of these are private adoptions that are instigated by the birth mother seeking help, and the other half are public, resulting from court-mandated removal of children from the birth mother's custody (Child Welfare Information Gateway 2008).

Adoption, in parallel with medical treatment, usually entails hefty fees and extreme surveillance by outsiders—in this case, by licensed social workers and family court judges—who assess the potential parents' fitness (moral, social, financial, and physical) for raising children (with medically assisted conception, biological fitness is more meticulously examined and manipulated). However, adoption is in many ways qualitatively different from medically assisted routes to motherhood. Plenty of people who are neither childless nor infertile adopt children. Unlike ART-created children, adopted ones are more apt to be stigmatized because of suspicions about lack of prenatal care, in utero drug or alcohol exposure, attachment problems, the inheritance of birthparents' presumed innate inadequacies, and the presumed weakness of the emotional and kinship bonds between the children and their adoptive families. For some, this anticipated stigma trumps the "spoiled identity" (Greil 1991, after Goffman 1963) attributed to the infertility of the prospective parents. Thus, the fantasy about who is saving whom changes. In using ARTs, the newly created miracle babies save their parents from the stigma of childlessness and restore their normativity. Adopters, in contrast, are thought to save their adopted children from poverty, abuse, and reduced life chances, and sometimes even from governments with repressive gender ideologies like that of China.

Journalist Liza Mundy (2007, xv) writes, "The spectacle of someone trying to have a child can be more inflammatory than the spectacle of someone trying not to have one." In this statement Mundy recognizes the scrutiny of women charting alternative paths to motherhood as well as the controversial nature of ARTs. Several researchers (Greil 1997; Lasker and Borg 1994; Becker 2000; Inhorn et al. 2009; May 1995) note that infertile women seeking motherhood face financial barriers, stressful medical procedures, psychological effects, lack of reliable information, moral and religious dilemmas, legal questions, and threats to personal relationships. Despite these difficulties, women will go to great lengths to become mothers if the cultural imperative is sufficiently strong, the medical procedures promising and comfortingly routinized, the success stories frequent and hope inspiring, and the desire to mother persistent and prolonged.

These women are in the minority among infertile women. When last measured in 1995, just 44 percent of white women diagnosed with infertility sought any medical treatment (not just high-tech versions); only 31 percent of their African American counterparts did so (CDC 1997). A tiny percentage of these two groups attempt adoption in order to become mothers (Fisher 2003). More recent statistics on all childless women (not just infertile diagnosed) show a general decline in the use of infertility services (12 percent of women in 2010 versus 16 percent in 1995) (CDC 2012). We know from the analysis of survey data that class, race, income, age, marital status, and education factor into who forges ahead with infertility treatment and who does not (Stephen and Chandra 2000), but the reasons for these distinctions are less clear. It appears that among African American and Latino infertile women, indirect reasons like social cues count more toward the differences in treatment access than the related variables of income, education, and health insurance coverage (Greil et al., "Race/Ethnicity," 2011). This book explores some of these emergent, indirect reasons.

2

CONCEIVING STRATIFICATION

And when Rachel saw that she bore Jacob no children,
Rachel envied her sister; and said unto Jacob, give me
children, or else I die.
—*Genesis 30:1, King James Bible*

Procreation is a fact of life. Actually, it is *the* fact of life. Infertility, then, can be confounding, albeit in different ways. For example, the stigma of infertility is so strong in Ireland that couples stay silent on the matter, making it seem as if the condition does not even exist (Allison 2011). Poor Egyptian brides find themselves outcast and prey to those who would sell them snake-oil cures if they do not give birth to a son soon after marriage (Inhorn 2000). In China the one-child-only rule morphs into a virtual one-child mandatory policy for women dealing with infertility (Handwerker 2000). And it could mean the "infertility treadmill" of repeated failures of IVF treatment for middle-class American women faced with the life-course disruption of infertility (Harwood 2007).

Infertile and childless women arrive there via unique pathways based on their individual lives. But the historical, political, social, and cultural context always colors the experience. In the United States, as in most of the world, motherhood is assumed to be part of the normal life course, and this assumption deeply affects infertile and involuntarily childless women (Pfeffer 1993). At the same time, childlessness is an allowable choice with many proponents. Whether or not childlessness is voluntary may not always matter to the experience of it (see McQuillan et al. 2012). The ever-expansive reach of medicalization, with the monitoring and manipulation of women's procreative bodies in particular (Turner 1995 [1987]), however, reinscribes the old mother-hood mandate with a new twist. Infertility, advancing age, or lack of a male partner need not stop a woman from making babies; there are always improving treatment options as well as alterna-tives like surrogacy and adoption. Marginalized women experi-ence this pronatalism differently, depending on their positions, in ways both oppressive and surprisingly emancipatory.

Getting the Message

The views, attitudes, and behaviors of marginalized women with infertility or involuntary childlessness reflect different histories (Ginsburg and Rapp 1995; Greil et al., "Race/Ethnicity," 2011; Lewin 1993). American pronatalism has its roots in patriarchal Abrahamic tradition and an agrarian past. Infertility among the Puritans was seen as a punishment for religious lapses, and worldly interventions like herbal remedies were not permitted (May 1995). The pathologizing of poor women's motherhood, by contrast, already existed in colonial times, as servant women could be turned out of the household for becoming pregnant.

Beginning with the late-eighteenth-century Revolution and continuing into the era of Manifest Destiny, American whites— rich and poor alike—contributed to the project of nation build-ing by having many children. The idea that an important reason to have children was to bring happiness to their parents grew in popularity at this time (May 1995). The "cult of true woman-hood" characterized women as rightfully dedicated mothers (Welter 1966).

But true womanhood was only meant for some. Native Americans suffered from the genocidal result of westward progress and the loss of children to assimilation projects like the "orphan trains" that stopped at frontier outposts to supply childless white families with workers/heirs. Enslaved African American women were valued less as mothers than as breeders and as capable nurses and caring "mammies" to white children, sacrificing their opportunities to mother their own children (Davis 1981). Meanwhile, Chinese women, first brought overseas to serve as prostitutes or house slaves—known as Mui Tsais—were treated as commodities, forcibly sterilized, and often prevented from marrying or reuniting with their spouses (Silliman et al. 2004; Yung 1995).

Dramatic social change in Victorian times up until World War II included the rise of the companionate family, responsible for "fulfilling the emotional and psychological needs of its members," replacing, for the middle class at least, the kind of traditional family that was tasked primarily with providing education, economic security, and social welfare (Mintz and Kellogg 1988, 108). Among whites, having children was considered a civic virtue and children were greatly sentimentalized.

Despite the "race suicide" panic that called on white Protestants to stop shirking their civic duty and propagate their race, 20 percent of women in 1920 were childless, the highest rate ever recorded. Attempts at social engineering—which included outlawing abortion for fear that white women were using it too much—largely failed, although eugenic ideas and worries about immigrant birthrates settled themselves into the American consciousness.

The postwar Baby Boom subdued the cries of race suicide. Children as a national obsession was clinched, however, and the family was seen as a haven from outside pressures (May 1995). This pronatalism was less a call to action and more a hegemonic practice: 95 percent of women said they intended to have children (May 1995). Everybody was doing it.

During the subsequent women's movement that challenged mid-century conformity, calling for an end to patriarchy and imperative motherhood, some participants turned the mandate on its head. These "earth mothers" extolled a *matriarchal* future that idealized motherhood and constructed it as the ultimate expression of womanhood in a way that rejected patriarchal conventions and parenting norms (Hartsock 1983; Ruddick 1989; see Thompson 2002). The uptick in lesbian and queer parenting today echoes this challenge; "mothering" can be enacted by any gender and in a way that creates families (and, ostensibly, new young citizens) who subvert the status quo (Stacey 2011).

By the 1950s infertility and childlessness came to be considered more personal tragedy than evidence of witchcraft, moral shortcomings, or malingering; and nonmotherhood is still seen by most as a sad a turn of events for a woman. American core values include the beliefs that all American married couples should reproduce and should want to do so (Veevers 1972, 1980). The importance of motherhood among women diagnosed as infertile happens along a continuum (Greil and McQuillan 2010). For women going through infertility—and some are "okay either way" in terms of motherhood or nonmotherhood (McQuillan et al. 2011)—the experience varies.

Poor women, Latinas, and African American women are more likely than other US women to begin motherhood before marriage, often at younger ages and before they have reached financial stability (Anderson 1999; Edin and Kefalas 2005). Communities cut off from educational and economic opportunity may value motherhood more highly in some ways; young women achieve adult status not via college graduation, marriage, or career advancement but as mothers. Poor women and women of color, then, may expect to begin having children at younger ages. Mainstream discourses, on the other hand, pathologize teen pregnancy and what is seen as profligate, "unplanned" parenthood, a concept that may not even be salient to low-income women (Barrett and Wellings 2002). Certainly many Latinas, who tend to be Catholic, forgo contraception as part of their religious practice, making family planning (in the precise way middle-class white couples usually think of it) less relevant. The Latino culture of *marianismo* glorifies mothers and motherhood. Some Latinas and members of other minority groups (like Arab American women contending with different kinds of patriarchy, pronatalism, and Islamic strictures against certain treatment) who cannot get pregnant experience intense stress over their frustrated motherhood (Inhorn et al. 2009).

Single women and lesbians, especially those who are well educated and middle class, are subject to greater social pressure to have children now that it is technologically possible and now that there are some legal safeguards (Agigian 2004; Johnson 2009) A number of actors and social forces construct the "normal gay," who pursues goals like marriage and parenthood that parallel the norms of straight society (Seidman 2004), and this profamily movement in the queer community has gained momentum (Stacey 1996, 2011). Older women, too, are bombarded with the notion that it is not too late to have children. Images of celebrities in their forties displaying their pregnancies are common. And news stories about older mothers (e.g., grandmothers carrying their daughter's future babies) pop up regularly. Cultural messages specific to certain groups (race/ethnicity, age, sexual identity, marital status) have to be understood as partial because these women are both insiders and outsiders. That is, infertile and childless women across the social spectrum hear and evaluate, resist and accept, popular ideas about motherhood and nonmotherhood as well as the messages within their own communities. It is important to remember that even with the promotherhood messages that get handed down in different ways to different groups of women, most infertile and childless women seek no remedy. The history and current status of childlessness in America is a closely related but separate aspect to the story.

Without Child

The stigma of childlessness waned with the widespread availability of birth control and abortion, and the women's movement and the sexual revolution improved women's procreative control in the 1970s. Childfree living was a viable option, one promoted by some feminists, by lesbians on the heels of the 1969 Stonewall Rebellion (see Stacey 1996), and by environmentalists worried about the population boom. Women could pursue other life interests and careers instead of being burdened with the task of raising children. Infertile women and the involuntarily childless became virtually indistinguishable from those who intentionally declined motherhood; thus, until medicalization intensified with the advent of ARTs, childlessness was less likely to be seen as pathological. Divorce was more common and women married later, trends than continue to inch upward. There are more than twice as many voluntarily childless women (7 percent) in the United States now than there were in 1982, and these women have always had the lowest religiosity, the highest income, and the most prior work experience when compared to other groups of women (Abma and Martinez 2006).

Even with cultural changes, suspicion persisted about the character and potential negative social impact of women who could make the choice not to have children (Blake 1979; Calhoun and Selby 1980; McAllister 1998; Miall 1994; Morell 1994, 2000). The phrase "choosing childless" makes it sound like women purposefully select that status. In fact, most childless women—even those who identify as voluntarily childless—do not. Many childless women can be described as "perpetual postponers," who make several short-term decisions that affect delays in family building until the end of their fertile years (Bulcroft and Teachman 2004; Heaton et al. 1997; Houseknecht 1987; Kneale and Joshi 2008; Zabin et al. 2000). Sometimes circumstance makes women childless, and sometimes they do "choose" it but only in the context of multiple life events (Carmichael and Whittaker 2007; Chancey and Dumais 2009; Kemkes-Grottenthaler 2003). Tellingly, researchers in one study were surprised to discover that one-third of their involuntarily childless participants (as identified by the researchers) later claimed to be intentionally childfree (Jeffries and Konnert 2002).

Some of those identifying as childfree by choice can be viewed as "wavering noes" (Morrel 2000), as these women hold out the possibility of having children if circumstances align differently. They may change partners and have a change of heart as well (Zabin et al. 2000). Just as women resist labeling their pregnancies as "intended" or "unintended" (Moos et al. 1997), childless women may reevaluate their intentions to fit their actual lives. A coworker of mine in her sixties once told me with a shrug that she "must not have really wanted" children or else she would have had them. Some women simply insist that they lack the so-called maternal instinct, and this self-perception obviously plays into decision making but does not preclude later, perhaps unintentional, pregnancies or eventual step-motherhood (Park 2006).

Whether the childlessness was voluntary or not, older (permanently childless) women are not necessarily bereft (Alexander et al. 1992; Letherby 2002b; Zhang and Hayward 2001). A couple of decades ago, childless seniors had fewer emotional ties and less help (Koropeckyj-Cox 2002). Increasingly, however, childless men and women who develop and sustain social networks and those who immerse themselves in work and leisure activities report satisfaction with their lives (Koropeckyj-Cox et al., "Women of the 1950s," 2007; Parry 2005; Pollet and Dunbar 20008; Slagsvold et al. 2009). In fact, it may be that childlessness is primarily a stressor in young adult life (McQuillan et al. 2003), perhaps limited to one's time in treatment (Becker 2000). Either way, well-being with respect to childlessness and infertility is mitigated by many factors in people's lives, ranging from class, race, and age to family attitudes and the quality of social support (Exley and Letherby 2001; Greil et al., "Variation," 2011; Umberson et al. 2010). Some voluntarily childless women boast a liberated attitude in which despite the "disbelief, disregard, and [accusations of] deviance" (Gillespie 2000, 223) that they put up with in their social interactions, the women are unapologetic and regularly deflect attacks on their femininity (mainly by attending to feminine dress and makeup or to the selfless nurturing of pets) (Slagsvold et al. 2009). Defying stereotype, many childless-by-choice women see themselves not as career-oriented feminists but as reasonable people concerned about the responsibility and financial burden of having children (McAllister and Clarke 1998).

Ideas about families are changing dramatically right now. Conventional American attitudes about childlessness may be going the way of the once-widespread opposition to same-sex marriage. A Pew Research Center survey and census figures reveal that in 2008 close to half of Americans (46 percent) viewed women's childlessness as making no difference in the expected quality of their lives (Livingston and Cohn 2010). This percentage has been creeping upward for decades, and a couple of smaller studies suggest that majorities of college-age

Americans view lifetime childlessness favorably (Koropeckyj-Cox et al., "Through the Lenses," 2007). The motherhood mandate may be weakening significantly. The medicalization of infertility interrupts this trend.

Fixing Infertiles

Infertility is a medical problem as well as a women's problem (Mies 1987). Medicalization places natural processes under the purview of medical authority. Just like other functions and states of women's bodies including menstruation, pregnancy, and menopause, medicalization of infertility and childlessness tells us that these statuses need expert monitoring (Lock 2007; Simonds 2002; Turner 1995 [1987]). At one time, infertility was but ill fortune. Now popular culture, the websites and literature for fertility clinics, and ads for fertility pharmaceuticals remind us that modern medicine can make miracles happen. This was not always the case under medicalization.

One physician lamented in 1920, "There is still, I am sorry to say, a tendency on the part of many general practitioners to recommend a little 'stretching and scraping' to every disappointed bride who comes to them (Child [1920] quoted in May 1995, 76). Doctors wanted to help these women and they still do.

Although a few doctors in the United States were running clinics as early as the 1940s (Marsh and Ronner 2008), women experiencing involuntary childlessness had little medical recourse; medical treatments were still more likely to render women permanently infertile than to help them (Marsh and Ronner 1996). Until the end of the Victorian era, men were thought to be fertile as long as they were not impotent. The eventual realization that gonorrhea and other conditions could reduce sperm production soon led to insemination techniques, including donor insemination (Moore 2007). At first, women could order self-help books and kits to accomplish insemination, but public dissent and the professionalization of medicine put a stop to that freedom.

Doctors may have felt they could not refuse women who "demanded" infertility treatment even if there was little likelihood of success from the procedures available (Marsh and Ronner 1996). An ethnographic study of infertile American couples in the mid-1980s found that women whose class status was equal to or greater than that of their doctors tended to demand treatments even with little promise of success (Greil 1991).

On the other hand, doctors' fiscal attraction to the lucrative emerging business in fertility, as well as their efforts to make their reputations by exercising their newly acquired expertise, played a role in the rise of infertility treatment (May 1995; Spar 2006). For their part, childless women, including single women, were for a time encouraged to adopt from the overflowing children's homes. By 1920, however, baby shortages were the norm, and the emerging adoption establishment began to weed out the unworthy from the pool of prospective adopters, further pushing women toward medical solutions.

Research picked up the pace significantly, and in 1951 medical practitioners in the United States started the journal *Fertility and Sterility* to facilitate progress in surgical techniques and pharmaceutical solutions. By 1970 drug manufacturers introduced hormonal drugs—namely Pergonal and Clomid—that could induce ovulation and promote pregnancy for many previously infertile women. The landmark 1978 birth of Louise Brown, the first "test-tube baby," created via in vitro fertilization opened the floodgates to a soon-to-be thriving infertility industry. The 1980s "me decade," saw a sharp rise in consumerism and the pursuit of individual satisfaction. Fittingly, fertility clinics offered a service for the well-to-do consumer/prospective mother who was seen as wanting a child to better her enjoyment of life. Feminist observers, though, viewed the broadening of infertility services as potential instruments for greater patriarchal control in terms of the ideology of compulsory motherhood and of direct manipulation of women's bodies (Mies 1987; Klein and Rowland 1989; Rapp 1988; Rothman 2000b; Solomon 1989; Sandelowski 1991).

And the flipside of popular cheerleading for medical advancements like IVF—a distinctive technophilia and interest in progress permeated public attitudes throughout the Cold War—was a moralistic distaste for women who had been career building when they should have been family building. The abortion debate peaked at this time, facilitating the rise of the Christian Right and the Moral Majority, evangelical Christians who equated "traditional family values" with male-headed households that included a wife and devoted mother who was the antithesis of the strident, bra-burning feminist. Yet at the same time, invoking both the promise of science and the grace of God, media stories abounded of medical miracles in which infertile or childless women could suddenly become mothers thanks to IVF and related procedures or perhaps via surrogacy. This media fascination helped usher in a new era of pronatalism.

The fertility industry and its consumers successfully mainstreamed the procedures by cleverly couching these technologies in the language of "choice." The use of private funding streams instead of federal grants in developing IVF and the like shielded these technological interventions from moral reprisals until well after the spread in usage (Marsh and Ronner 1996). Patients' higher social status as married, white, and middle class in the early, more selective years of ART further protected it from the kind of criticism that might lead to restrictive policies. There were highly publicized kinks, however.

The Baby M case, in which Mary Beth Whitehead, a surrogate mother, refused to give up the child she was contracted to bear, unleashed a backlash. Some advocated for the maternal bond created in pregnancy. Others, revealing long-standing class tensions about good and bad mothers, found her less worthy as a parent (and untrustworthy since she had reneged on her contract) than the wealthier couple who hired her to have *their* baby. Many commentators privileged the husband's genetic tie (he provided the sperm) over that of the surrogate (she provided both the eggs and the womb). Elizabeth Stern, the childless woman who hired the surrogate, had not been shown to be infertile; rather, she had been told that pregnancy could exacerbate her multiple sclerosis symptoms. This fact bothered many commentators who thought she should have tried to get pregnant first.

The arguments revealed a distrust of women's ability to make sound procreative decisions (May 1995). This case prompted feminist social scientists to draw connections between attacks on abortion and the growing prevalence of infertility treatment (see, for example, Rothman 2000b). Antichoice advocates and popular and medical perspectives on ARTs ideologically separated women from their eggs, fetuses, and embryos. The rights of women are further separated from the rights of their fetuses through the proliferation of prenatal testing, fetal surgery, and the arrests and imprisonment of drug-using pregnant women (Casper 1998; Morgan and Michaels, 1999; Rapp 1999; Simonds et al. 2007; Thompson 2002). Observers criticize the simultaneous commodification and personification of embryos and fetuses (Morgan 2006) and the false promises of "embodied progress" that elevated technological advancement at the expense of women's claims to their own bodies (Franklin 1997). But these criticisms could do little to slow down medicalization of infertility.

Lobbying by medical interests helped steer legislation toward increasing medicalization. For example, the medical community pushed for greater access to IVF treatment via mandatory insurance coverage. The fertility clinics, exposed in the 1980s for providing misleading statistics—some clinics accomplished no "successful" pregnancies—backed the federal Fertility Clinic Success Rate and Certification Act of 1992. This law charged the Centers for Disease Control (CDC) in Atlanta with compiling statistics on IVF volunteered from the approximately 483 fertility clinics in existence nationwide. The move was part regulation, part marketing strategy (Spar 2006).

Medically assisted conception continues to increase with the advent of more refined technologies. Screening of cryopreserved semen extended from HIV monitoring to routine testing for a host of genetic diseases and anomalies. Contemporary ART options include not only IVF facilitated by ovulation drugs but also egg donation, embryo donation, gamete intrafallopian transfer (GIFT), zygote intrafallopian transfer (ZIFT), intracytoplasmic sperm injection (ICSI), and testicular sperm extraction (TESE). Clinics cultivate relationships with gestational surrogates and solicit egg donors to round out the catalog of treatment options.

In general, the new technologies up the stakes for infertile and childless women and men. The mere availability of options compels women to try treatments (Franklin 1997) even when they may be ambivalent about motherhood in the first place (Mundy 2007). It is simplistic and a bit patronizing to suggest that women are merely duped into their interest in ARTs (cf. Chodorow 1978; Crowe 1985), but ARTs certainly increase pronatalist social pressures (Agigian 2004; Harwood 2007; Sandelowski 1991). Women encountering infertility often experience "bodily disruption," the condition in which the betrayal of one's body must be overcome, usually via a medical "journey" (Becker 2000). Becoming a mother heals infertile women, and puts their lives back on the right track. At the same time, the rampant medicalization of procreation (Greil 1991) and the industrialization of reproduction, as Adele Clarke (1998) describes it, or "Infertility, Inc." (Mamo 2007), helped build the image of the medicalized, consumer-oriented, and driven Infertile Woman, who remains a slightly pitiable and accursed figure. An alternative future narrative would broaden the acceptable roles for women so that infertile women could choose treatment or not without undue social pressure (Ulrich and Weatherall 2000).

Stratified Infertility

The *fertility* of poor women and women of color is constructed as a social problem but their *infertility* is not (Davis 1981; Lewin 1993). Race, for instance, makes a difference whether a woman is valued or devalued as a mother, or whether her children are considered precious or a burden on society (Roberts 1997; Rothman 2000b). As medical ethicist Alan Meisel explained when asked what the medical profession was doing about class (and race) disparities in infertility care, "[obtaining] the essentials in life for one's own health is more crucial than the possibility of creating more people" (quoted in Rotstein 1997). In this framing it is nearly unfathomable that poor women would suffer from infertility. The system of "stratified reproduction" (Ginsburg and Rapp 1995) means that structural inequalities severely constrain procreative choices for women at or near the bottom rungs of the social hierarchy (see also Dworkin 1983; Roberts 1997). Created under colonialism, racism, sexism, and homophobia, this system persists.

When studying procreative technologies, it is vital to ask "who *uses* them and who gets *used* by them" (Klawiter 1990, 84). Late in the nineteenth century, physicians began to carry out a significant program of reproductive surgery and experimentation on poor African American women and immigrants (Marsh and

Ronner 1996). Disenfranchised women seeking medical attention became unwitting study subjects as medical experimenters gradually learned from poor women's bodies how to treat "mechanical" and hormonal imbalances among apparently infertile middle- and upper-class women, culminating in the first in vitro experiments in the 1930s.

Some poor women sought medical treatment for infertility, usually in the form of insemination (Marsh and Ronner 1996), but many more poor women and women of color found themselves sterilized—often just after a hospital birth—without their permission (Roberts 1997). In the early decades of the twentieth century, compulsory and coerced sterilization began in prisons and mental hospitals and extended to public maternity wards and public health service clinics. These programs did not cease completely until the mid-1980s (Roberts 1997). Unfortunately, this tendency to disregard the reproductive rights of marginalized women continues. In July 2013 California lawmakers called for an investigation into allegations that inmates in California state prisons had been sterilized—sometimes even coerced—without proper medical approval and oversight. Arguably, providing experimental birth control drugs and devices —and even undue pressure to use safe contraceptives—in low-cost clinics in recent years constitutes de facto sterilization as well (Davis 1998; Roberts 1997). With the arrival of AIDS and the ensuing rush to assign blame, poor women's and African American and Latina women's fertility problems were more likely to be attributed by health practitioners to sexually transmitted infections than to the treatable, fertility-threatening condition of endometriosis (Nelson 2003; Nsiah-Jefferson and Hall 1989). This widespread misdiagnosis increased the prevalence of infertility among these groups (Ferre Institute 2001).

Even before the first successes with frozen embryos and surrogate mothers, Angela Y. Davis (1981) presciently described a dystopia in which some women would be classified as "breeders," making babies for the benefit of the elite. This standpoint complicates the utopian vision held by some white feminists who thought perhaps that pregnancy and childbirth could be removed from the woman's body, taking place in a laboratory and thus freeing women from those procreative chores (Firestone 1970). Davis's less sanguine predictions have come true both in America and globally. Thirty percent or more of gestational carriers are black women carrying the genetic progeny of white couples; the race difference aids in the construction of the surrogates as mere incubators, not related to the fetuses they nurture and deliver with their bodies (Ragone 2000). They are the modern-day equivalent to the wet nurse whose job was classified as another kind of manual labor. Impoverished women in India can now earn the equivalent of several years' salary by acting as commercial surrogates for Westerners' frozen embryos, which they "hand back" after birth (Associated Press, 2007).

Essentialist attitudes about genetics privilege the creation of white babies and white families while casting families of color as inherently inferior, an ideological trend documented in the contexts of transracial adoption, interracial surrogacy, and interracial families (who are seen as misfits) (Twine 2000; Gailey 2000; Ragone 2000; Rothman 2000a; Duster 2003). The 1965 Moynihan Report, officially titled *The Negro Family: The Case for National Action*, reflected and produced white attitudes and governmental policies regarding black families, lamenting the high fertility rate of African American women and maintaining that "at the center of the tangle of pathology is the weakness of the family structure" (31). Foster care and adoption from poor families to better-off ones were thought to help break the "cycle of poverty" and later, to rescue so-called "crack babies." I know from my own experience with public adoption of "drug-exposed" babies that this reasoning is still very much alive.

The image of hyperfertile Latinas also erects a rhetorical barrier against procreative freedom. It precipitates divisive legislation such as California's voter-approved Proposition 187, which sought to deny social services, including education and health care, to the children of undocumented immigrants. Supporters of such laws claim that Mexican women enter the United States in alarming numbers to give birth to "anchor babies," whose care would require plundering public coffers. Federal courts found the California law unconstitutional, but the sentiment and legislative actions persist nationwide.

Stratified reproduction affects economically marginalized whites, too. A concerted effort ensued throughout the twentieth century to search out, find, and remove children from "feeble-minded" (a proxy for lower-class) parents and to subsequently place them with "good families" (May 1995; Marsh and Ronner 1996; Fessler 2006). Lower- or working-class women in the United States experiencing infertility or involuntary childlessness must contend with this tenacious prejudice. In England, where public fertility clinics treat working-class patients and offer the back-up plan of adoption to those who do not complete a pregnancy via ARTs, "victim blaming" and disqualifying home studies appear to be standard conduct on the part of the authorities (Monach 1993). In the United States, poor women often cannot get help for infertility (nor, paradoxically, abortions) via state health programs, but they can get sterilized for free. Indirect barriers to treatment for poor and working-class women may be more significant even than financial difficulties; it can be especially difficult to make it to doctors' appointments during the workday if one has an hourly wage job, for example (Bell 2009, 2010).

Lack of interest in assisted procreation among African

Americans and Latinos originates with individual cues (e.g., interest in parenthood) and social cues (like family encouragement), but a large portion of the variance between whites accessing treatment and these other groups is as yet unexplained (Greil et al. 2009). Some economically marginalized racial and ethnic minorities who do pursue treatment struggle to pay for medications and ARTs (Inhorn et al. 2009), but statistical investigations show that this frustration does not fully account for why most do not seek help (Greil et al. 2009). There is a misguided tendency on the part of some medical gatekeepers to blame the minorities' "cultures"—which are judged to be overly religious or patriarchal—for their disinterest in fertility treatment, but this explanation has not held up to scrutiny (Culley 2009). There are varying levels of comfort and facility with doctors' authority and with medicalization in what Thompson (2005) calls "biomedical citizenship" and Mamo (2007) calls "cultural health capital." As Rayna Rapp (1999) explains in her study of amniocentesis, less privileged women with limited science education—a group disproportionately composed of poor women of color—tend to "get off the conveyor belt" of medical surveillance early on. They fear what they do not understand, commonly misinterpreting medical jargon and the language surrounding statistical probabilities.

Minorities and the poor are not only less likely to seek medical cures for infertility but also less likely to be adoptive parents. The National Association of Black Social Workers, alarmed at the rate at which black children were being taken and placed in white homes, strenuously objected in its "Position Statement on Trans-Racial Adoption," disseminated in 1972. The organization then readdressed this issue in the 1991 "Preserving African American Families" and 2003 "Preserving Families of African Ancestry" position papers, which called for more more African American adoptive families and greater respect for informal adoption among kin and community members; yet whites still account for 90 percent of prospective adoptive families. Marginalized women cannot experience infertility or childlessness without respect to the inherited American system of stratified reproduction. They can, however, sometimes turn the situation to their advantage.

Emancipatory Stratification

More single women and lesbians access infertility treatment (and adoption) than ever before. Although stratified reproduction negatively impacts these women and calls their fitness for motherhood into question, the increase in single motherhood, medical ethics committees' recommendations, and a need for more customers opened ART and run-of-the-mill assisted-conception techniques (donor insemination) to these groups (especially for those who are also white and/or middle class). Single motherhood by choice is increasingly common and increasingly socially acceptable—even expected in the absence of an appropriate romantic relationship in which to raise children (Klett-Davies 2007). Arguably the heterosexual use of ARTs and adoption help normalize those avenues toward parenthood for gays and lesbians (Park 2006).

A lesbian baby boom began in the 1990s. No longer did women need to choose between life outside the proverbial closet or motherhood: gay women assumed they could have both. Fertility clinics offered anonymity, safety measures like screening semen for infectious disease, and other services (e.g., choice in donors, legal safeguards, and even sex selection in a few cases). For these reasons, fewer lesbians restrict their procreative attempts to the low-tech techniques of home insemination than they once did and now employ hybrid strategies that combine high-tech medicalized fixes and the low-tech do-it-yourself techniques (Mamo 2007). They can take advantage of these means of procreation while also enjoying the benefits of their outsider sexual-identity status (Agigian 2004; Haraway 1991). Many enjoy a special sense of community and belonging, heightened credibility in a social justice milieu, and consequently some freedom from traditional norms and mores. Still, obstinate barriers and fertility clinics' subtle discrimination slow full-scale participation in these procedures by lesbians and single women (Johnson 2009). Religiously affiliated clinics may turn them away; single women and lesbians have less income than married couples and thus less money for treatments; and clinic language can be alienating by assuming clients will be accompanied by their husbands.

The women of *Not Trying*, these less medicalized and socially marginalized infertile and childless women, hear the conflicting messages that motherhood is a social imperative, yet suspect for some groups of women that childlessness yields both stigma and freedom, that medicine meant for yuppies can fix their infertility as well. Stratified reproduction as it happens in America provides the backdrop to their individual experiences, but they take every opportunity to pick and choose as needed from the various narratives about motherhood and nonmotherhood to make sense of their own lives as infertile or childless women.

3

MOTHERHOOD FROM THE MARGINS

> A woman who can bear children is held in higher
> esteem than a woman who cannot. The culture
> is, or used to be, very harsh on people who could
> not bear children. Because once you're married,
> your job is to have kids. It's just that you're a baby-
> making machine. So if you cannot have them, it's
> like, "What is wrong with you?" —*Annie Adoyo, thirty,*
> *second-generation African immigrant, single, student*

Women can be single, childless, professionals, artists, healers,
nuns, and workers; but they are also mothers a priori, imbued
by society with a maternal femininity. In their book *Pregnant
Pictures*, Matthews and Wexler (2000, 2) posit, "Most women
must deal at some point in their lives with the possibility, im-
possibility, or fact of becoming pregnant." This understate-
ment—for I would argue that virtually all women encounter
these facts several times in their lives—goes for motherhood
as well.

Most of the twenty-five women I interviewed for this study
do not fit within what Dorothy Smith (1993) calls the Standard
North American Family (SNAF), an ideological code akin to
DNA that defines family, the basic unit that forms society. The
SNAF family consists of a household that includes a mascu-

line father who does most of the earning, a feminine mother/ housewife, and their biological children. Beyond the reduced code of SNAF, the ideal family variant (or dominant allele, to continue Smith's DNA analogy) is presumed white and middle class. The participants in this study represent a cross-section of women who are childless or dealing with primary or secondary infertility—designated as less essentially feminine—who also belong to social groups that mainstream society portrays as dubious candidates for motherhood anyway: women of color, poor women, lesbians, and single women.

I further describe them based on their reasons for childlessness. Feminist poet and scholar Adrienne Rich (1976, 250–51) offers insight:

> There are women (like Ruth Benedict) who have tried
> to have children and could not. The causes may range
> from a husband's unacknowledged infertility to signals of
> refusal sent out from her cerebral cortex. A woman may
> have looked at the lives of women with children and have
> felt that, given the circumstances of motherhood, she
> must remain childless if she is to pursue any other hopes
> or aims. . . . A young girl may have lived in horror of her
> mother's child-worn existence and told herself, once and
> for all, *No, not for me.* A lesbian may have gone through
> abortions in early relationships with men, love children,
> yet still feel her life too insecure to take on the grilling of
> an adoption or the responsibility of an artificial pregnancy.
> A woman who has chosen celibacy may feel her decision
> entails a life without children. Ironically, it is precisely the
> institution of motherhood, which in an era of birth con-
> trol, has influenced women against becoming mothers. It
> is simply too hypocritical, too exploitative of mothers and
> children, too oppressive.

The study interviews reflect a similar range of motivations and circumstances. These less medicalized women's reported experiences reveal that there are multiple pathways to involuntary childlessness/infertility (statuses that are, in fact, fluid). Two are *childfree by choice*, both college-educated lesbians in their fifties who display second-wave feminist sensibilities: they see motherhood as a trap designed to subjugate women. The three young, low-income, urban African American women are childless because of an *intentional delay*. They differ from their older sisters and aunts as well as their peers, siblings, and cousins by putting off pregnancy—and serious romantic relationships—to pursue education and get a foothold on a career. These young women depart from the expectations others have for them and instead embrace mainstream values about the proper life-course trajectory, a plan they are able to follow, they say, thanks to material support from their families and "God's will." A few women—the ones who are *potentially ready*—still hope to become pregnant should the perfect conditions present themselves. They are all three single, self-supporting women over thirty, and two of them have minimal involvement in any children's lives.

Childlessness "just happened" for quite a few of the women. Other life events intervened and diverted their attention. Two of these women are close to menopause and have not yet ruled out pregnancy—and both are exploring adoption—but they differ from the *never readies* in that they appear to be willing to identify as nonmothers if adoption does not pan out. The *infertile identified* includes women who unsuccessfully tried to get pregnant and then pursued medical help. This interface with the medical industrial complex—with doctors, nurses, specialists, laboratory technicians, pharmacists, and counselors—medicalized them. That is to say, the experience probably altered their perspectives, leading them to more closely identify with the status of infertile. These infertile-identified women, all of whom are married or engaged, include those who never birthed a child and those who had one and then were told (or realized) that they could not or should not have any more. It is significant that none of these women are absolutely, 100 percent certain that they cannot, or could not before menopause, become pregnant and bear children. That is, they mention that they have or have had some opportunity to achieve pregnancy. Four adopted a child (and two of these are currently fostering an additional child with the hope that it will lead to adoption); three say that they have accepted that they will only have one; and just one is still pursuing medical help. Finally, one woman, Robin Smith, a counselor for a fertility clinic, can be described as *de facto infertile*. Robin, like many other lesbians and like some single women, was seeking, at the time of the interview, "alternative insemination," in Amy Agigian's (2004) usage, and taking fertility drugs to improve the probability of success.

Real Moms, Bad Mothers, and Other-than-Mothers

> *The "childless woman" and the "mother" are a false polarity, which has served the institutions both of motherhood and heterosexuality.*
> —Adrienne Rich, *Of Woman Born*

When asked about what it means to be a woman, nearly all these women—across lines of race, class, age, sexual identity, and marital status—talk about one's capacity for motherhood, whether or not she was a mother herself:

> Although of course not all women are mothers, most have the potential to be. And that makes us very different from men, just having that. Most people I see tend to be closer to their mothers than their fathers. Even if the relationship

can be difficult, there's a different bond. . . . Part of being a woman is being a mother. —*Aikiko Moto, forty-three, Japanese American, married, secondary infertility, teacher*

Women have that responsibility in terms of bearing children. It's not something you can pass off to the men. I also feel that in general in our society, women have a bit of elevation or respect because they are capable of that. Especially these days, with the sperm bank, I think men realize, I hope, that women don't need them as much perhaps. —*Emily Reilly, thirty, white, single, fast food restaurant manager*

I think it's a beautiful thing to be a woman because we are the ones that give life. We're the ones that give life, carry life. We're like a miracle within, I think. And, I think being a woman is a gift as well as a miracle. And, I'd rather be a woman, than a man. [*Laughs*]

Kristin Wilson: Why?

Just because we are able to do that. Maybe not so much in my case. But at least our body, the way we are built, we are supposed to be able to do this. So, I think that in most is what to me is being a woman. Now that I'm older, I see it that way. —*Lupe Jimenez, forty-one, Latina, married, electronics technician*

These passages reflect the paradigm of the maternal body as fundamental to the social body. Aikiko emphasizes the maternal bond as the basic social relationship; Emily views the use of sperm banks as liberating women from men; and Lupe's comments show that merely the *potentiality* to "give life" essentializes women as mothers. Lupe's own childlessness challenges the very definition she gives. A female body that is nonmaternal can cause loss of feminine identity:

> I found out [the infertility diagnosis] through this specialist in San Francisco and he was an older man and it was just horrible. It was just this older man saying, "Well, you can never have any children." . . . And of course I'm sixteen. I'm like [*makes a blank face*], "Okay." Like no questions; I just like, boom, totally shut down. And, then, I didn't feel like a woman. —*Jessie Silva, forty-two, white, queer, hairstylist*

> Without my uterus, even though I went through a lot [of pain and medical procedures], I wouldn't feel like I'm a woman. So I'd rather keep it. That why I left it [contrary to medical advice]. —*Zara Senai, forty-five, African immigrant, married, laboratory technician*

Each of these women negotiate a new, strained relationship with her disorderly maternal body while they also negotiate with the men who control—and attempt to normalize—those bodies with surgery and medicine (see Britt 2001); Jessie, as a powerless teenager, "shuts down," refusing to interact, whereas Zara insists on keeping her uterus, an organ that is both problematic (prone to cysts in her case) and the keystone to her embodied womanhood. Jessie repeats throughout her interview that taking pills to bring on menstruation made her feel "less of a woman." She finally stops her daily doses after a couple of decades, perhaps not coincidentally at just about the same time that she redefines womanhood with the aid of self-help seminars and a pagan-inspired women's circle she attends each full moon. The healing was possible, and necessary, but it was slow because she felt betrayed by what she felt was her nonmaternal, unfeminine body. Still, many women oppose this narrative:

> I have the utmost respect for single parents, you know, but I think some women really feel like they just have to have a baby because they're a woman, and I just said, "You know what? Whatever you feel, but that is not right."
> —*Penny Ortiz, fifty-two, Latina, single, guidance counselor*

> I think for a woman sometimes it is to the peak to be a female and be a woman once you give birth to a child. Personally, it is not the way I think. . . . They say [incredulously], "You don't have kids?" It's like I should have a kid to be a woman. And I don't see it that way myself. I always was afraid in my life of two things: that I will be a prostitute or a drug addict. Those things were a panic for me. And why? I don't know. But I would say, "How miserable will my life be if I get pregnant? My dad will kick me out of the house. I will be on the streets with a child with me." Those things were in my mind. And maybe that is why I always thought to have a child would be a big responsibility for me, that I was not capable. But recently when I said I am not married and I don't have kids, people suddenly look at me and say, "You're fifty-six and never got married? You are fifty-six and never had kids?" But I see it like they are questioning my sexuality.
> —*Lourdes Garcia, fifty-six, Latina, single, office assistant*

Both Penny and Lourdes are outspoken women in their postmenopausal fifties, childless, single, and satisfied with their lives. They belong to the group for whom nonmotherhood "just happened." Their critiques of the motherhood mandate help them resolve any lingering doubts and strengthen their identities as fully complete women despite their childlessness. These two women, Latinas whose mothers modeled social expectations by having many children, already distinguish themselves by having careers and—for Lourdes—by wearing pants and not wearing make-up. This pants-wearing metaphor has long been used to make fun of wives who assert themselves—and the hen-pecked husbands who allow it. Lourdes constructs her pants wearing as an expression of her freedom from a patriarchal family and culture. She notes that others often question her sexuality because she does not have children. Yet she is self-accepting and defiantly a woman.

Like Lourdes, many of the women locate themselves and others along a continuum that connects femininity, motherhood, and womanhood. I propose a way to visualize their constructions as a series of concentric circles with the "real mom" at the center, a woman who performs her "natural" role by being nurturing, self-sacrificing, and loving. By virtue of their feminine praxis, women with biological children, as well as those with formally or informally adopted children, may fit this description. Outside the nucleus is an outer ring corresponding to a secondary type of mother: the "nominal mother," who may not have planned her pregnancy and who lacks the means or emotional resources to care properly for her children, but who is still seen as feminine and womanly to the extent that she fulfilled her biological destiny. This (straw) woman—whose shortcomings help define the "real moms" by contrast—fails to hear her calling and does not fully inhabit motherhood. The nominal mother is analogous to the "bad mother." The next ring signifies the "godmother auntie," a woman who does not achieve womanhood from having children herself but who is not childless. She exercises maternality in her intimate involvement in the lives of her nieces and nephews or godchildren, for whom she provides advice, financial support, and childcare.

Finally, we can imagine the outer ring, on the periphery of all the others, as the "less involved nonmother," a woman who self-reports nonmaternal traits like selfishness or an intolerance for children and who does not have children in her life to any substantial degree. These categories are not exclusive ones, and an individual woman may self-identify—or may label others—differently, depending on the temporal and social context.

In an absurd contradiction, motherhood is seen as honorable and central to womanhood, while the day-to-day work involved—the mothering—garners little respect or material support from society. The women I interviewed expressed a spectrum of views on motherhood, some based on an idealized—rather than an experiential—vision of mothers.

REAL MOMS

I either asked directly or probed each woman I interviewed for her thoughts on what makes someone a mother, a question frequently interpreted by the woman to mean, *What makes someone a good mother?* Some women offered, in a rote manner, little more than predictable lists of virtues such as "patient," "listener," "loving," "forgiving," "selfless," and "comforting"; others told me that the mother is the core or glue of the household or family. A few called up more specific, if hypothetical, images that portray mothers—and themselves—as feminine nurturers:

> I had always pictured that I would be a mother and I even pictured myself making big bowls of bread from scratch with the yeast and rolling it out, and making big bowls of soup. So I always pictured myself as a mother with kids.
> —*Dianne Jacobsen, fifty-eight, white, divorced, life coach*

Several respondents measure a good mother by her ability to produce quality children—by whatever means:

Being a mother means unconditional love, nurturance, protection, and guidance and teaching. If you're a good mother. How to be a decent human being and grow up with ethics and morals, and just raise somebody phenomenal who could contribute to society maybe, or just be a nice person contributing to society, making the earth a nice place. —*Talia Stein, forty-one, white, single, home healthcare aide*

Children are like animals. They will do whatever they can get away with. And if you don't enforce that line, they will overstep whatever boundaries you think you've set. . . . Communication [is also important to being a good mother]. I think my mom was a great mom. We were definitely disciplined. We knew those boundaries were there. I got spanked a few times. I know some people don't believe in spanking but I am not entirely against spanking, because like I said, little children are like little dogs, and they need a little smack. —*Annie Adoyo, thirty, second-generation African immigrant, single, student*

You sort of have to give them everything: love and support and kindness and encouragement. And yet not be overprotective or pushy or anything like that. I think you have to find a good balance between being really supportive and loving, but also firm. I think my friends and my sister-in-law are incredible mothers. All my friends have been really good. I can see that my friends' kids have confidence in themselves, but none of them are bratty or act out. It's sort of a balancing act between being really there for them but allowing them to be independent at the same time. —*Karen Tabb, forty-nine, white, single, teacher*

Beginning with choosing a partner or sperm donor, mother-hood is something of a eugenic enterprise. The social reproduction of "good values" is an extension of this emphasis on quality. For Talia, Annie, and Karen, a mother's task is to pre-ternaturally draw on her intrinsic motherliness—to nurture and to guide—in perfect balance. The converse to this valorized task of dedicated, purposeful, self-denying childrearing is the long-standing tradition in Western society of blaming mothers for their children's flaws and crimes (see Ladd-Taylor and Umansky, 1998; May 1995; Chodorow 1978). The three women quoted above are all childless and have yet to confront the reality of this ideal mothering. However, just the social knowledge that mothering is supposed to entail a full immersion—a baptism and reawakening as wholly different women who "give everything"—affects their plans for pursuing that role.

In their definitions of "mother," some of the women emphasize the hypothetical practicalities involved in mothering, using phrases like "financially stable," "provider," "orderly," and "organized" to describe what being a mother means. These women equate motherhood with work, both inside the home and outside it (because of the financial demands of having children). Their views range from seeing motherhood and its attendant responsibilities as difficult but laudable and indicative of maturity and goodness to believing it to be a bad choice that reveals meager personal integrity:

> I always thought of having children as a way to
> completely give up your own needs, and your own goals,
> and direction in life. . . . It's way too much work to be a
> mother. . . . I saw my mother as kind of a slave really. She
> worked constantly raising kids. —*Lana Marks, fifty-two,*
> *white, lesbian, nurse*

I can honestly say [my teenaged cousin is] trying. . . .
She goes to work. Picks her son up from daycare. Comes
home. She cooks, cleans. A real mother. Her life is gone.
Well, not gone, but she can't do half the things she wants
to do because of her son. She never says he's a burden,
but she says sometimes she gets frustrated and tired to
where she can't take it. —*Jamilah Washington, nineteen,
African American, single, student*

One, let me start off by saying, it's a blessing to be a
mother. I believe it takes someone who has a lot in them:
patience, love. To see after someone else and put them
before yourself, put their needs before your needs, and
their wants. It's a pretty big task. . . . It's a job. It's a really
big task. And it never ends really. . . . I don't think it's
possible to be a mother and not be warmhearted and
take responsibility. I don't even know the word for that.
But I don't think it's possible to be a mother and not do
those things. Because if you're not doing any of those
things, what purpose are you serving? —*Nicole Lambert,
twenty, African American, single, student*

Lana's view of motherhood as drudgery and limiting contrasts
with Jamilah's subtle admiration of her cousin's earned designation as a real mother. Annette Kramer, a fifty-four-year-old
lesbian, talks about her awe of intentional mothers who will
strive to do it better than their own mothers. For Lana, motherhood is not a role any self-actualized woman would want.
Both Lana and Annette are childfree by choice in a sense and
middle-class lesbians who came of age during women's liberation—long before the so-called gayby boom—when conventional roles for women were being rejected. Neither has had
children in their lives much since adulthood, perhaps because

they cast off wholesale these roles and embraced an alternative lifestyle but probably also because they were aware of the distrust society has had for gay adults in relation to children. They see motherhood as an undesirable experience, not something they would miss. By contrast, Jamilah and Nicole, who represent a group of women who enact an intentional delay, hail from poor communities in Oakland, California, and recognize motherhood as an acceptable reality of adulthood, a phase they are not yet ready to enter. Though both young women repeatedly point out that their peers have all had children already—and thereby have already entered adulthood, a pattern documented by sociologist Elijah Anderson (1999) among other inner-city African American adolescent girls (see also Edin and Kefalas 2005)—their primary definition of motherhood as work steers them away from taking it on too soon. A more experiential take on both the emotional aspects and the mundane practicalities of motherhood comes, quite expectedly, from the mothers, all of whom were identified as infertile at some point in their lives and thus have ample impetus to ponder these meanings:

Kristin Wilson: What does it mean to be a mother?

It's a big responsibility. Let me tell you. I cannot sleep in anymore because he will wake up at six o'clock in the morning and either ask me for a bottle or ask me to watch *Sesame Street* at six o'clock in the morning. . . . he wakes up really early and is a big responsibility. It means that I have somebody to take care of and that I have somebody that might be able to take care of me when I grow old. —*Serena Lopez, thirty-nine, Latina, married, pharmacy technician*

It's wonderful. Our baby is—she's so sweet. It's a lot different than I thought it would be. It's more all-consuming of your life than you think it's going to be. You kind of think it's going to be this thing like on the side. It's really like it becomes your life and suddenly other things are not that important. Like at my work, I was trying really hard to like get promoted, move up the ladder and all this stuff, and now suddenly I don't really care. I just want to do my time, do my hours as early in the morning as possible, leave as soon as I can so I can get home with the baby. —*Jennifer West, forty-six, Latina, married, engineer*

If probed on the difficulties of motherhood or on the emotional rewards, respectively, Jennifer and Serena would agree with Aikiko Moto, a forty-three-year-old teacher, who describes motherhood as equally hard work and unfettered joy. But when just asked what it means to be a mother, their initial reactions are revealing. Class differences between the two may partly explain their differing descriptions of motherhood. Whereas Hannah Johanson, a thirty-nine-year-old part-time teacher, who enjoys adjustable work hours and a husband who shares more equally in the childcare, marvels at the emotional rewards of motherhood, Serena, who has a more conventional marriage wherein she works the "second shift" and bears the lion's share of childcare duties, fixates on the responsibility involved. Motherhood for Serena is toil and sacrifice (and old-age insurance); for Hannah it is achievement and personal happiness. Jennifer, who once doggedly competed for promotions in a male-dominated profession, feels indifferent now, transforming her identity (temporarily?) by refocusing her energies to her newly adopted baby. Their experiences, though perhaps a little surprising to them in their magnitude (e.g., their universal shock at the amount of laundry), are expected and largely defined by social class.

Mothering for all these women for whom motherhood came about only with difficulty means subsuming themselves into society's idea of what a mother is supposed to be. Yet mothering can be seen and experienced as more adult responsibility and less warm and fuzzy bonding, depending on where a woman is situated in this stratified society. This truth that is so clear to the young black women I interviewed, women who have seen their peers struggle to be proper mothers, is obscured in society's fantasy of motherhood, an image held by some infertile and childless women. Infertile and childless women are thought to desperately want to be mothers, specifically the kind of mothers for whom childcare "becomes [one's] life." But an acknowledgment of the disparities in women's economic and social situations is not usually part of that narrative.

Not only are there very different day-to-day realities between groups of mothers on the basis of structural factors, but there are also unique histories and attitudes. Australian sociologist Christine Everingham (1994) argues persuasively that mothering— as socially constructed, not driven by innate responses—involves women asserting their own needs and interests (like affection and status). They are themselves agentic "subjects": they do not just learn to respond to babies' cues in culturally appropriate ways but negotiate their needs with the perceived needs of their children, and not every action is instrumental in intent (Habermas 1990). Such women as Hannah, Serena, and Jennifer, who pursue motherhood in the face of multiple obstacles, exercise their agency in service of their own needs and interests. Yes, motherhood is expected of them, but this is not the only reason why they become mothers. We must also discard that tenacious trope—still promoted in the medical and psychological literature—that instinct drives women. They balance their own desires—desires that are not entirely socially determined (but also not instinct-driven) as appropriate to their social positions.

Tellingly, some of the respondents bring up the concept of ownership in defining what it is to be a mother:

> Joy, love, those are the best words I can describe it with. The happiness that I have with my son. The happiness is so fulfilling, so fulfilling. When I think of my son, I just smile. I just have to see his face in my mind and he makes me so happy. Even though, I mean, all kids have their days, but just knowing that he's mine, it makes me feel like I have won. —*Lupe Jimenez, forty-one, Latina, married, electronics technician*

> I guess to feel completed in life and, yes, this baby is making me really, really happy in every way. Sometimes I can't stand him but, yes, he makes me happy, so I believe in having somebody that belongs to me. This baby belongs to me. It's really nice. —*Serena Lopez, thirty-nine, Latina, married, pharmacy technician*

Lupe, who suffered a couple of miscarriages first, then went through a difficult pregnancy before birthing a one-pound, fifteen-ounce premature son, feels as if she has won a prize. Serena, a mother with secondary infertility and only hypothetically considering adoption, sees motherhood as a completed life goal and expresses some characteristic (for her) ambivalence about her satisfaction with motherhood ("Sometimes I can't stand him . . ."). She chooses to emphasize ownership of her baby. It is noteworthy that she uses the term "belong" here, a word that means not only ownership but also implies fitting in and can also indicate the natural order of things. All meanings apply. The baby and Serena belong together as mother and child, belong to one another in the primary human relationship; and the baby belongs to Serena, as Lupe's belongs to her—as in their personal property. It is revealing, incidentally, that Serena does not use the term "us" to include her husband as a co-owner. To her, children are extensions first and foremost of the mothers, entities whose purpose is to make their mothers happy and fulfilled (and to make their fathers proud); they are not quite full persons in their own right. Both of these women describe an initial period of terrible disappointment at their secondary infertility, and they indicate a redoubling of their attentions on their singleton children, a situation that may increase possessiveness. It is common, nonetheless, to refer to one's *own* children, suggesting that ownership is an integral characteristic of the relationship. Having one's own children is preferable to adoption or to other close relationships with children, for example.

In a capitalist society in which property ownership symbolizes individual autonomy, the ownership of children implies that rearing them is a private venture, not a public one. This attitude creates tensions with doctors, teachers, neighbors, social workers, law enforcement, and relatives who all claim some responsibility in seeing to it that children are raised in accordance with societal values. This surveillance more significantly affects poor women and women of color, who are more likely to lose children to the system. Maybe Lupe and Serena, both women who have witnessed—albeit at some distance—children being taken by the state, feel the need to establish the permanence of their mother-child relationship by stressing ownership.

Another description of a good mother—what I term a "real mom"—that emerges in several of the interviews is "being there":

> What makes a good mom is being there for their kids. Being there for them in whatever they want. Since my parents are divorced, my mom was always there for me and my brother. Even today, we are both of us grown and

we have our own families and she is always there for us, you know. [*Sighs*] . . . Being a good mom is not easy, but it's a job for life. And we'll be kids all the time even when I'm fifty and my mom's seventy; I'll be a kid for my mom. I want to be my mom really; I want to be like my mother. She was divorced when she was thirty years old; she was never remarried. She never really wanted to meet anyone else, which is not good. She concentrated on me and my brother to be where we are right now. If my mom wasn't like that, we wouldn't be here. . . . I mean 80 percent of the time, if the kids are coming from a family or loving mom, those kids are most likely to have their own family [reflect that]. —*Azra Alic, thirty, Bosnian immigrant, engaged, apartment manager*

I'm not that close to my mom. We don't have that perfect mother-daughter relationship. We do talk and she helps me out and things like that but we don't have that special bond like that. But I'm going to have that with my child. I've learned from things of my parents' past. One thing you don't do is favoritism . . . If you do, keep that to yourself. And you know always be there for your child and so like that. —*LaWanda Jackson, forty-two, African American, single, nursing assistant*

"Being there" connotes a permanent, lifetime commitment in which women prioritize above all else their roles as mothers. These ideal mothers dedicate themselves physically and emotionally to their children, and as Azra indicates, ensure the social reproduction of family-oriented values. Mothers or nonmothers, middle class or working class, black or white—women who fit all these categories emphasize being there. Obviously, a mother's success or failure at "being there" is subjective. Its meaning can vary from lending a sympathetic ear to sacrificing one's romantic life to supporting a child long past adulthood. The thesis of Sharon Hays's *The Cultural Contradictions of Motherhood* (1998) is that good mothers must be intensive mothers whether or not they work outside the home. Infertile and childless women grasp this directive, and depending in part on their circumstances, they may imagine this life as gratifying, terrifying, or some combination of the two extremes. Working-class women and women of color see ideal mothering as providing direction, discipline, basic necessities, love, and permanence; the white, middle-class model of mothering can seem to them neurotic and overbearing. Although their precise understandings of real moms differs, one fact is certain: the focus on mothers accomplished at being there contrasts sharply with those other mothers constructed as hapless, unready, and unavailable.

NOMINAL MOTHERS

Mothers cannot escape the incessant public scrutiny of their work. Infertile and childless women chime in as well. To wit, many of the interviewees volunteered parables about hypothetical and particular bad mothers:

> One of my nieces was with her mom in Sacramento, and I went to pick her up and on the way home she just poured her heart out. . . . She said, "You know my mother used to call me a bitch since I was three years old?" She said, "I can remember that. She still calls me a bitch." And I said, "You know that is so sad to me because a mother shouldn't even be using that kind of language to her children. A mother shows love. A mother shows respect because that's how you learn." —*Penny Ortiz, fifty-two, Latina, single, guidance counselor*

[This follows a story about a friend who had a baby to (unsuccessfully) "keep a man."] I don't want to say lesson, because I don't want to say, "You having a baby is your punishment." But that was a lesson, something she had to learn. You're being selfish because you're only thinking about this man. You don't think about bringing a life into the world! And you have to take care of that baby whether he is in your life or not. . . . I hope she's taking care of the baby. I really do. Sometimes you have a baby and you don't even care about it. . . . It's kind of like, "I have you, but what good are you now?" And then you drop the baby off on family members, and that's not fair to the baby! The baby didn't ask to be here, and the baby doesn't deserve that kind of treatment. —*Nicole Lambert, twenty, African American, single, student*

These kinds of comments reflect societal fears about negative social reproduction, or those cycles of poverty or bad living that produce women who have children but who do not behave like "real moms." Molly Ladd-Taylor and Lauri Umansky (1998, 2) explain: "Some mothers are not good mothers. No one can deny that. There are women who neglect their children, abuse them, or fail to provide them with proper psychological nurturance. But throughout the twentieth century, the label of 'bad' mother has been applied to far more women than those whose actions would warrant the names. By virtue of race, class, age, marital status, sexual orientation, and numerous other factors, millions of American mothers have been deemed substandard."

Infertile and childless women of all backgrounds grapple with this concept of the nominal mother, who represents an inferior kind of woman who, despite her immorality, is still assigned higher status in terms of womanhood than they are thanks to a technicality. Blaming mothers accomplishes many nefarious goals. It provides societal scapegoats, allows others to define themselves more favorably against their opposite, serves an allegorical function, boosts divisive political rhetoric, represses women, maintains existing social hierarchies, and ensures social reproduction. The sexual minorities (especially the lesbians), women of color, and single women I talked with occupy categories that would automatically make them "bad mothers" in the eyes of many. Thus, these women have to preemptively intervene in this discourse to deflect the future label of "bad" or nominal mothers from themselves. A general attitude lingers that childlessness indicates punishment for gender-role transgressions. Just as in the Protestant ethic, wherein those called by God can be identified by others in their receipt of many blessings, so too are mothers assumed to be God's chosen. It is this context in which the infertile and childless women point their fingers the other way, toward those women who—through some cosmic mistake—became mothers but do not deserve that status.

Nominal mothers sometimes came up when a woman wanted to point out the unfairness of her own difficulty in having children:

> I hated anybody that had more than two children; I
> mean I hated them. I would despise anybody that had
> more than two children. I hated the fact that women
> that didn't deserve children would have them. . . . I felt
> I was treated so unfairly in life because I knew I could be
> a great mother to other children. And that's why it hurt
> because I just felt that I could do it. My husband and I
> are financially okay and we would be great parents and
> why weren't we blessed? What did we do in our past? I
> felt that we were being punished. What did we do in our
> past that this was happening to us? —*Lupe Jimenez, forty-
> one, Latina, married, electronics technician*

In this way of thinking, why should those who refuse to heed the "being there" prescription, who, for lack of character or maturity are financially unstable, be rewarded while the truly deserving are inexplicably punished? Lupe tells me also that she began to lose her religious faith precisely because of this dilemma. Some of the mothers in this study contrasted their reasons for having a child with some of the more selfish reasons they imagined others to have:

> Some people would like to have children because it's a way of continuing the species, one of them. Pass on what they've learned. I think kids are lots of fun and they bring a lot more love to your family and your home. I think some people do it for more selfish reasons, and I think some do it without thinking about it, unfortunately. So there could be parents who are parents, but it's more like they are biologically based rather than doing the actual work.
> —*Aikiko Moto, forty-three, Japanese American, married, teacher*

Aikiko, who (consciously) talks more generally of parents, rather than just of mothers, emphasizes that these so-called parents—who *could* exist, but who are not real people she knows—refuse to do the "actual work" of parenting, the work being essential to the definition of parent. It is telling that she uses the term "parent." As with the word "mother," it functions as either a noun or a verb. One who biologically reproduces yet does not do the work is called a "parent" or a "mother," but others like Aikiko, lacking a word to describe these less than parents, must content themselves with knowing that these reproducers are not really parents. In American slang usage, the term "sperm donor" now means any uninvolved or estranged father, not just one who donated to a sperm bank. These men may *father* a child by contributing male gametes, but they do not *parent*. There does not appear to be an analogous term for a mother who does not mother, as its meaning is oversaturated.

Although society generally perceives "bad" mothers through the lens of prejudice (i.e., mothers who are racial or ethnic minorities, teenagers, impoverished, single, and sexual minorities), sometimes bad mothers can occupy privileged social strata:

> I have this girlfriend who spent over $100,000 trying to get pregnant. She'd fly from Palm Beach through Atlanta over to Alabama to get artificially inseminated every month. When she came to Atlanta, she'd try another technique; she'd stay at the Ritz. What she wanted to do is—she had a doctorate, she had a law degree, everything she wanted, she'd always had, and this she couldn't get. So she was willing to go bust out anything. . . . But she ended up marrying. She ended up going to MENSA, a guy in the MENSA society for years. He was the biggest drag in the world. He had no personality at all. But she wanted to be with him so they would have smart kids. Then she decided to go with a jock. I went through four marriages with her, and she had already been married before and she was after that elusive thing. But she wouldn't have known what to do with a baby, with a child. She just wanted to get pregnant and have that baby. —*Dianne Jacobsen, fifty-six, white, single, life coach*

Dianne, an infertile-identified adoptive mother, taps into critiques of consumerism, eugenics, careerism, and instrumentalism. Her friend exemplifies the calculating businesswoman for whom children are highly commodified and represent nothing more than the opportunity to put another feather in her cap.

In contrast to Dianne, who subsists on a limited budget, this wealthy woman seeks bragging rights instead of a mutual, loving relationship.

The notion of nominal mothers helps childless and infertile women situate themselves in a comfortable place within the schema of motherliness/femininity. Their infertility or childlessness places them outside standard notions of womanliness; and by placing some mothers in a spectrum as inferior to others, they dissociate being a woman from being a mother, a classification that can range from merely giving birth and—in unmammalian fashion, returning immediately to one's own self-interested pursuits—to all-consuming devotion. They typically emulate or admire the real moms on their pedestals—even if they cannot envision themselves in that role—and regardless of their own status as mothers, godmother aunties, or less involved nonmothers, they place themselves above the nominal mothers.

Nominal mothers are thought to be too selfish to fully immerse themselves in motherhood. These fallen women's perceived lack of planning and assumed lesser emotional investment are unforgivable in the eyes of many of the women I interviewed. The working-class women and the women of color tend to point more to the cycle of poverty and the perpetual immaturity of the mothers as the most unfortunate outcomes of nominal motherhood, whereas the white and/or middle-class women lament the dearth of "wantedness" and the injustice of easy fertility for the unappreciative and less deserving. In concert with political pundits and everyday bigotry, they demonize and blame a faceless bunch of women for societal ills, but the irony is that the stereotypes are usually culled from prejudices about the very groups to which many of my respondents belong: the poor, working-class, African American, Latina, immigrant, and lesbian communities. This fact merely increases their need to distance themselves from these unacceptable mothers.

I love those two kids. I don't know what love means when you have your own child, how could I love more someone else? I mean, really love those kids and they love me and I'm their aunt and I—I just don't know how much I can love someone else when I have a lot of love for those two kids. —*Azra Alic, thirty, Bosnian immigrant, engaged, apartment manager*

Azra, the only woman pursuing IVF and one of the most emotionally invested in having her "own" children (at the time of the interview), describes the deep love of what I call a "godmother auntie." The label refers to the voluntary role—sometimes under considerable pressure—taken on by women who have close relationships with others' children. The godmother auntie can be distinguished from an "aunt," a mere title imposed from the cultural kinship system, or "godparent," sometimes an insubstantial, ritual designation. Godmother aunties also differ from aunts who raise their sibling's or friend's children, as I would classify these as adoptive mothers who may belong in the real mom category.

Fully half the women I interviewed call themselves aunties and/or godmothers. They animatedly, and proudly, describe the godmother auntie as one who loves unconditionally, who keeps alive family traditions, who purchases tickets to special events, who finances vacations and "extras," who provides guidance, who joyfully babysits, who teaches about volunteerism and other moral values, who listens without judgment, who provides an escape from abusive parents, and who generally "spoils" the children. But her role and status differ from those of real or nominal mothers. Though she may feel an abiding love for the children, she is always at some remove from them and from that perfect feminine status enjoyed by the "real moms." Stepmothers may fit into this role or they may more closely fit the role of "real moms," depending on the intensity, quality, and extent of their relationships with their stepchildren. Some of the women detail their long-term—even intergenerational—roles as especially involved godmother aunties:

> My niece, the twenty-six-year-old, she's my goddaughter. When she was eighteen, she got pregnant and she said I was such a good godmother to her that she wanted me to be the godmother of her daughter. . . . And, I love those babies. I love them so much. And it's nice because when they see me they—there is so much love . . . they are jumping on me and I love it. "Give me more hugs, more kisses, you know I love it." [*Speaks animatedly*] I'm the only one when I leave that my nieces and my nephews come to kiss me. . . . So there is just a real special bond with all of them. I guess when they were little, I didn't have any kids and so I always used to pick them up and take them to Toys"R"Us and take them to the movies. And it was like rent-a-kid. And I loved being with them. I absolutely love being with all my nieces and nephews. And, they wanted to go and tell their secrets to [me] and they would talk to me before they would talk to their parents. —*Lupe Jimenez, forty-one, Latina, married, electronics technician*

> I think it was God's calling for me not to be a mom, you know. I love being an auntie. And you know how people say, "Oh yeah, because you can just take them all day and then dump them back with their parents?" I never think that. . . . And I have some traditions that I do with nieces and nephews. And they wait for me to do them. . . . I remember one of my little nephews came over and he said, "Auntie"—he's looking around; he's been there

for a while and they would just come over. . . . "Auntie, do you have any little children?" And I said, "No." And then the other one said, "Well, why not?" And I said, "If I did, I wouldn't get to spend all my money on you guys. I wouldn't be able to take you out on vacations. I wouldn't get to buy you some new shoes." "Oh" he says, "I like that." He's the older one. So they, I think, grew up thinking that big women have little children. Isn't that weird? I thought that when he said that to me. And then that I mean the aunt is just like freedom. I would've never—I don't know what I would've done with my own children. Would they have traveled like my nieces and nephews? Would they get what I've given these kids? I don't know, I don't know what it would be like. But I have felt free to do [for them].

—*Penny Ortiz, fifty-two, Latina, single, guidance counselor*

The godmother auntie connotes a special bond as well as freedom. This role enables women to love, nurture, and enjoy children—and to provide for them in selfless ways—but at the same time the giving does not require giving up much. Penny has the "freedom" to provide financially and emotionally for her nieces and nephews, the freedom to limit what she provides, and the freedom to do what she wants to with her life. This role does not completely satisfy Lupe, but it does satisfy Penny, suggesting that a social theory of infertility or nonmotherhood must account not just for blithe, childfree living but also for otherhood roles in which children are decidedly significant. Jamilah further explains how being a godmother auntie can be enough:

> I wouldn't say that everyone should [have a child]. I know of people that are satisfied. Like my best friend, her little sister, her godmother, she's satisfied with just being a godmother. She can get them what she wants. She takes

care of them just like she was their mother. Helps them, supports them in school. She asks their mom, "What do they need so I can help them with that?" or "Send them down to me." Things like that. Matter of fact, they find comfort in her more than their own mother. "Oh, I want Godmother. I want Godmother." She comes to them. She don't feel that. She doesn't feel that. She'll tell me, "If I'm supposed to have kids, God will give me kids in time. But for now I'm content with what I have." She's almost forty. She's content. She says she don't have no wants right now as far as children. She says she's selfish. She don't want to give. And she know if they're her children, it's like she has to. I mean, her godchildren—she does for them. But it's not the state telling her she has to, or society is not saying, "Oh, you have to provide for your godchildren." Because I know lots of godmothers who don't do anything. —*Jamilah Washington, nineteen, African American, single, student*

Being a godmother auntie involves nurturing, an activity attributed to the nature of women. But these godmother aunties relate an experience that to some extent strains against discursive control. Although they enact the nurturing expected of women, they also do this nurturing much on their own terms. What they offer to children is not mandated by the state or by strict social convention, as Jamilah notes. Some aunts are distant relatives and some godmothers are just old friends of the children's parents. Those women who turn it into something special choose to do so each and every time they interact with the children. Being childless, as the above stories reveal, opens up an opportunity for women to enact a satisfying role that enhances their lives and the lives of the children they know. Based on these women's experiences, it does not appear that occupying the godmother auntie role is always a concession resulting from a frustrated desire for motherhood.

Nevertheless, since society exalts motherhood, some women who cherish and enjoy themselves as godmother aunties do not find it an adequate replacement:

> [My nieces and nephews] love me. Go over there and I can't even get them off my back. They call me Lalatiti. Lalatiti . . . that's like my little nickname. They love me and ask [*using child's voice*], "Lalatiti, when you coming over?" . . . They LOVE me. I'm a good auntie and I'm fun. I'm fun. One of my little nieces go . . . "Lalatiti, do you have a car? Do you have a car seat?" "Yes, I have a car seat." "Put it in back in my car so you can go with me." I said [*as to a child*], "You can't go with me." "Whyyyyyy?" She surprised me when she asked me that, you know. And I said, "One day I'm gonna have a child," and she say, "Noooo. I don't want you to have one. I want to be the only one." But it's a good feeling. Children know good people. Children are attracted to me. —*LaWanda Jackson, forty-two, African American, single, nursing assistant*

Jennifer West, a forty-six-year-old married civil engineer, talks about "borrowing" her nieces and nephews and being frustrated at having to return them to the parents' schedule. She and others mean to demonstrate through such comments that they are natural, capable nurturers. The godmother auntie relationship provides proof that the women are deserving of children, that they *should* be mothers, evidenced by the fact that children—who "know good people"—love them.

Women settle for this role even if they later revise its meaning as meant to be rather than as the default in the face of infertility and/or involuntary childlessness. The godmother aunties are in some ways better than real moms, and they certainly feel that they are better than nominal mothers. And yet they still view themselves as less than women because they do not have children of their own. In the Latina and African American communities, the auntie and the godmother roles have long been rooted in communal family life (reinforced by forcible separation during slavery and later through disproportionate imprisonment [Alexander 2012]). Thus, for the women with these origins, the status is recognizable and the duties are already partially defined. These roles exist among mainstream, middle-class whites, too, but they are less common and more likely to be superficial labels. Nonetheless, for all these groups there is a large measure of freedom encoded in this status. They can fully inhabit the role for a time or forever. It can be an outlet for their need to nurture, to feel connected, to take responsibility for children, to practice mothering skills, and to be recognized as feminine. Some turn the godmother auntie role into a master identity—occasionally pointing to length and depth of service as proof of their dedication and integration into a larger family—whereas others use it as a temporary stop on the way to motherhood.

LESS INVOLVED NONMOTHERS

About a third of the women with whom I talked were childless and described themselves as less involved in children's lives when compared to the mothers and the godmother aunties. Among the less involved nonmothers are a few different types: those who decline motherhood, those for whom childlessness just happened, and those who may still have children at some indistinct point in the future when they meet their personal, somewhat vague standards of readiness. Some declare their disinterest or allude to their self-perceived deficiencies as mother material:

> One thing is for sure: God is no fool. God would not give me a baby, I don't believe, not right now. Because I

don't have that much patience. I can watch them and the minute they wrack my nerves, goodbye! —*Nicole Lambert, twenty, African American, single, student*

In my early years, actually, I thought to have children placed a big, big responsibility. Maybe that's why I never thought about it, to have children, because I thought I was not capable; I didn't have the intellectual ability or the education to educate a kid. . . . Actually, some of my friends at this point have adopted kids. Some of them actually, that's the advice they give me, "Why don't you adopt a kid?" but I'm of the idea that I don't feel capable of giving the attention and all of what a child requires. I like to be independent. I like to be free. I like to do whatever it pleases me to do. —*Lourdes Garcia, fifty-six, Latina, single, office assistant*

In our interview, Karen Tabb, a forty-nine-year-old teacher re-flecting on her singlehood and childlessness, tells me that she loves children and finds herself "very drawn to them" but that her fear of them as all-consuming responsibilities prevents her from ever becoming a mother. Lana Marks, a fifty-two-year-old lesbian nurse who describes herself as childfree by choice, is alone among the study participants in her utter lack of ambiv-alence about her childlessness, yet even she employs the com-mon joke about the joy of having children around—for a little while. She enjoys her time with them, and unlike the godmother aunties, she also looks forward to giving them back. The less in-volved nonmothers often portray themselves—mostly without apology—as selfish in not wanting to devote every second of their lives to children. This counternarrative of fulfillment out-side the maternal sphere is possible post–women's lib, but it does carry a social cost:

It's natural instinct to want your own. . . . People who don't
want children [*in another voice*]: "I don't want no kids. I
don't want no children." It might be experience they may
have went through or they might just be selfish. . . . It's up
to them. I'm not there to question them, "Why don't you
want no children?" So it's like they own little reason . . .
some people say, "I'm too selfish." I was really hurt when
they say, "I'm too selfish. I'm not ready to settle down. I
want to do this and do that." I be like, "Can I have your
eggs then? Give me your womb." —*LaWanda Jackson, forty-
two, African American, single, nursing assistant*

LaWanda's judgments illustrate several widely accepted ideas
about voluntary childlessness. She implies that women who
do not want children are unnatural, selfish, immature, waste-
ful, and ungrateful (for their potentially functioning eggs and
wombs). The less involved nonmothers, whether voluntarily
childless or not, turn these accusations in on themselves. Like
those people LaWanda quotes who say, "I'm too selfish," the
women inventory their own nonmaternal traits. Conversely,
they also echo one another in frequent mentions of their freedom. Without children they can pursue advanced education,
travel, stay out all night, do whatever they want to do. They con-
cede their selfishness but enjoy their liberty all the same.

But accusations of selfishness abound in these interviews, and
this blanket term obscures more complex motivations and phenomena. The women accuse nominal mothers of selfishness for
their supposed inattentiveness to their children. On some level,
the selfish label reflects the envious feelings of those who cannot have children so easily. The less involved nonmothers who
abstain from motherhood or delay it are not only selfishly independent but also *unselfish*, they say, since they refuse to have
children whom they would not sufficiently "want" or dote upon.

The sentiment of having "always wanted" children crops up repeatedly in the interviews. Several of the infertile-identified and adoptive mothers say this about themselves or about women they know. To have always wanted children indicates some predestination and a natural inclination toward motherhood; those who have not always wanted children are automatically assumed to have always been less suited for it. The phrase "always wanted" can also serve as an explanation for the desperation of women who try too hard to have a baby, a feeling attributed to others—not themselves. They suggest that women who have always wanted children just cannot let go of the goal of having them, regardless of the obstacles and costs. Some of the less involved nonmothers seem to think that their ambivalence about motherhood further proves their maternal shortcomings. It may also entail a bit of self-protection, wherein women who cannot come by motherhood easily reflect on their motivations and repeatedly remind themselves that they never really wanted children anyway.

Though they have no children and some may be nominal aunts at best, most still find significant ways to help with children's needs. I can offer many examples: Mary makes baby clothes in her spare time for friends' and neighbors' children. Talia's job involves full-time care of a fourteen-year-old severely disabled boy. Karen, who has children's drawings all over her living room floor left over from a recent young friend's visit, receives a call from a neighbor during our interview asking her to babysit for two small children while the mother runs to the grocery store. Gloria, who began considering adoption because her house was "too empty," cares for her adolescent brother until he recently moved out on his own.

Several of the less involved nonmothers have borne considerable responsibility for the care of younger family members at some point in their lives, sometimes during their own childhoods. It is possible that on some level these women feel they already did their time raising children (see Gregory 2007). Indeed, some of the older, adoptive mothers I talked with who recall similar responsibilities indicate that they delayed childbearing because they needed the opportunity to be free, sometimes inadvertently passing up their fertile years. A need or desire for the autonomy they did not have growing up, then, may also partly explain some women's choice to be childless. In any case, they may be less involved with children now, but they have not always been that way. This fact underscores the fluidity of these categories in individual women's lives.

Some of the less involved nonmothers specify how they may sustain a feminine, nurturing identity through practices that do not involve mothering. Annie Adoyo, a thirty-year-old student, imagines a job with children as an alternative to having them herself; and Zara Senai, a forty-five-year-old laboratory technician who expresses much sadness at her infertility, relates her and her husband's choice to buy books, send money, and provide the financing for her brother-in-law to build a house in the city back in Ethiopia so that her nieces and nephews can go to a better school. The social stigma (or, more to the point, the resulting negative effect on self-esteem) attached to childlessness may be allayed by their devotion to the care of pets, partners, friends, or elderly parents and by their working in professions seen as altruistic and requiring mothering-like talents like nursing, counseling, and teaching. Childless women may reassert one aspect of their femininity (caring/nurturing) by pointing to these kinds of proof of their "maternal instincts" or stereotypically feminine qualities (Kirkman 2001). To be clear, I do not propose that all women who opt out of motherhood must find other outlets for their "motherly" qualities—qualities that are no more natural to women than to men. Their behavior likely stems in large part from their socialization as girls, their need to identify as gendered women or to project that image, and the career tracks most open to women.

The less involved nonmothers who are singles and lesbians live what second-wave feminism envisioned as the emancipatory ideal: freedom from the private patriarchy of heterosexual marriage with children. A couple of them concur with this vision, but there are several other takes on this status of the less involved nonmother. Their status may also be read as the result of having chosen from other substantial life options. For several women in this category of less involved nonmothers, childlessness just happened as a result of the vagaries of life events. They embrace the status a bit less comfortably, choosing instead to "not think about it." The younger women, of course, often view themselves as only temporarily less involved nonmothers. For them it is an appropriate and acceptable life stage between childhood and adulthood. But for the postmenopausal women who have been less involved nonmothers for decades of adult life, it is a permanent situation. Some claim no regrets and others acknowledge intermittent disappointment in the turn their lives have taken. But all recognize that their lives as nonmothers challenge expectations, and they find that they must defend and explain themselves to others even while they go about living complete, rewarding lives in which they contribute to society. They do not have to be viewed as stymied by childlessness or stumped by infertility, or as even the kind of women for whom being child-free is a badge of honor, an indicator of their feminist bona fides. Taking their claims of happiness at face value, one can see that their lives advocate a broader discourse about what womanhood means.

4

INDECISIONS

> People want children to be able to continue their
> bloodline. Psychologically, it gives you some sense of
> fulfillment. As human beings, you go to school, you grow
> up, you get a job, and you start a family. And you retire,
> and you go senile, and then you die. Finding a partner
> and starting a family is supposed to fulfill you.
> —*Gloria Owusu, thirty-eight years old, African American,
> single, project manager*

Gloria succinctly—if a bit cynically—outlines the standard life
course in US society. But when it comes to the part about starting a family, the women I talked with all found themselves off
that course to one degree or another, at times intentionally and
at times by circumstance.

Prior to beginning this study, I naively assumed that many
women made a definite decision to have children or not. Because
I thought that women who, like me, did not have children would
know whether or not they wanted them, I diligently crafted questions and probes for my interview schedule that were designed
to explore how these decisions were made: who influenced the
respondents, what kinds of reactions their decisions provoked,
what advantages and disadvantages they considered, what feelings surrounded their decisions. I quickly discovered that instead

of offering clarity, many of the women I interviewed would wa-ver in their answers. Some display greater ease in telling me first why "other people" want children, only later explaining their own reasons for wanting them or not. A few talk about having always wanted children, but at times even these same women con-template the negative consequences of having children, harbor doubts about their capabilities as prospective mothers, and de-fer to what many describe as God's unique plan for them. The women I interviewed often discuss motherhood as a basic, essen-tial function, the key to life fulfillment, for (other) women even while approaching the role a bit more cautiously themselves. They tend to be indecisive or simply unwilling to worry much about their own fertility and motherhood.

Motherhood Motivations

For many, motherhood is an expectation not to be questioned. My talks with women about why people have children and why they as individuals want(ed) or do not (or did not) want to have children, vary from general, philosophical musings to practical benefits and drawbacks of having children. Having children, preferably when "ready," provides the opportunity to fulfill per-sonal, biological, societal, or divine expectations, to ensure so-cial reproduction, and to enter adulthood.

Lourdes Garcia, a fifty-six-year-old office assistant, says that women exist on the planet to have and raise children. Similarly, Gloria Owusu acknowledges that having children is culturally prescribed, noting, "Children are like air . . . having children is like air. So everyone has children." Annette Kramer, a fifty-four-year-old family therapist, insists that many women have children without thinking about it. She claims that "it just sort of happens" and that yet, for some, motherhood is their *role* (her emphasis), meaning their calling in life, a calling they are helpless to ignore.

Motherhood can happen unintentionally—or, perhaps fortuitously—to a woman who goes on to fully embrace the role. Still, several women in this study remain dubious about this sequence of events. They often indicate that "most" people—not they—do not pause very long to consider their reasons for procreating. Infertile women and lesbians, for instance, do not usually have children as the result of a moment of passion. Their motherhood, if it is to happen at all, entails intention and clearing many hurdles along the way. This view sensitizes these women to careful consideration of motherhood, an attitude they expect of all good mothers, or "real moms." Mothers, in the abstract, are supposed to have "always wanted" children. However, the women themselves do not report having always wanted children, and this contradiction creates a tension in their self-understanding and their stories about why women become mothers.

The mothering instinct, the motherhood calling, and/or the need for the bodily experience of pregnancy and childbirth come up repeatedly as reasons why women might go to the trouble of pursuing motherhood. Several of the women indicate that pregnancy is the embodiment of womanhood. It is a tightly woven symbolic, physiological, and social experience. Many women assume it will happen to them and they want it to happen, and when it does not, they have to cope with the perceived loss of femininity. But there are options. Thirty-year-old Annie Adoyo hedges that her mothering instinct has "kinda, sorta come alive," leaving the logical door open for a different outcome. LaWanda Jackson, a forty-two-year-old nursing assistant, who wishes to adopt, says that birthing her child is important but not "that important," indicating that she is sad to let go of the bonding opportunity but, at the same time, as feminine experiences go, raising a child trumps birthing one. In fact, the adoptive mothers—generally busy with the daily responsibilities of childcare—barely lament the lost opportunity to carry a child and choose to expend little energy on regret. Emily, a new foster mother, still wants to experience pregnancy (she is looking into sperm banks); she emphasizes a social preoccupation with "collecting experiences." To her, motherhood enables personal growth. For others, motherhood can be a journey toward full womanhood:

> The reason why I want a child is—Well, now having one, I can grow in ways that I never thought imaginable and it makes me want to be the best person I can be having her. And she's the greatest teacher yet. —*Jessie Silva, forty-two, white, queer, hairstylist*

One grows as a person—as a woman—*through* the nurturing of a child. Nicole, from another standpoint, sees having a baby as motivating women to persevere. Being forced to grow up is the main consequence of motherhood in her view:

> I think a lot of the reason why people want children is to feel wanted, to feel that somebody needs me. To encourage them. If I have a baby, I have to go on for my child. I can't not work. I can't not continue on. I know that if I give up, then I'm not setting a good example for the child. And a lot of times it isn't planned. It's something that I think should be thought out before it happens. . . . I have a close friend and she has a baby. And the baby's father is in prison. But she didn't plan on having a baby. But when she found she was pregnant it was too late for an abortion . . . and we don't believe in abortions anyway. . . . I look at her as an example of what life would be like for me if I had a child. It's hard. . . . She's raising the baby alone . . . but the baby . . .

encourages her to keep going on. She is up at the crack of dawn going to work. She struggles just so she can make the money so that someone is there to watch the baby. — *Nicole Lambert, twenty, African American, single, student*

More privileged women than Nicole can set sight on the tender moments associated with motherhood:

I was very happy growing up and had a good home life and remember my childhood years as having been very happy ones, and so I wanted to share some of that. —*Hannah Johanson, thirty-nine, white, queer, married, teacher*

Though their backgrounds and perspectives differ widely, these women are not preoccupied with the goal of a baby or of the status of "mother," but with the process of mothering and the benefits of that process to themselves. I interpret this as a fairly emancipated perspective. These women are not in it (potentially) to fit in or to acquire a baby or to fulfill a directive of social reproduction; rather, they want the *experience* for its own sake (cf. Ginsburg 1989).

Having children also, according to the women I talked with, cures loneliness, theoretically brings one emotionally closer to a spouse, provides old-age insurance, is simply the result of a biological drive to reproduce, or is expected by God:

I have a lot of friends who have children because they feel that something is missing in their lives. They think a child will be able to replace that. —*Jamilah Washington, nineteen, African American, single, student*

I want a child because I was talking about how lonely I am. . . . I just been seeing if I want to adopt a child. Just a few weeks ago, I see on TV, *Calling All Angels,* and then about two weeks ago at my church, my pastor was like, "You know, a lot of children need to be adopted." And I was like, "Okay, God, I hear you." Because I was talking about all how lonely I am and waiting for that special husband to come along so I fixin' to say, "Okay, I hear you," and then that's how I ended up at the adoption agency. I feel that I could love a child; I have a lot of love to give. I'm patient. I'm experienced too. I work with children. I'm a nurse's assistant, so I work with children in pediatrics like that. And I handle like twelve babies, change their diaper and feeding them and rocking them and doing things like that in between other things that I do. And I'm the oldest of four girls so you know I have a lot of experience dealing with children. *—LaWanda Jackson, forty-two, African American, single, nursing assistant*

[People want children] because they want to have something in their life—it makes your life full I guess. I started thinking about like how would it be if we get old and we don't have any kids and also like how would it be if something happened to [my husband]? And he's my family. He's all I have and I didn't have any kids with him. I just felt like I'd be really lonely if I didn't have children. There's so many things that I'm into doing that I love sharing with children. . . . Like baking Christmas cookies each year, going to get the tree, making a big deal out of the holidays, and swimming in the tropics. *—Jennifer West, forty-six, Latina, married, engineer*

To be sure, the absence of someone to care for them in their later years is the only regret several of the women have about their childlessness. And this comment is often offered in jest.

To explain why some women do not have children, the women generate a much shorter list, one that mostly just adds negative dimensions to the themes explored above. Some women metaphorically shrug, saying that motherhood is not a calling for everyone. They have fewer narratives available to them to explain this deviance. However, several insist that one's life may already be full without children, or that some women lack the patience or commitment necessary, or that they themselves are not yet—or ever—"ready."

Readiness .

Readiness for motherhood is an important recurring theme in the discussions of fertility and infertility, childlessness, and transitions into motherhood. Readiness is a highly ambiguous concept that can change over time. It can mean being prepared in a practical way, having the correct social status (married and/or employed, for example), being emotionally and psychologically willing, or being primed biologically for motherhood.

Elizabeth Gregory's (2007) book *Ready*, based on interviews with fairly privileged professional women entering motherhood in their late thirties and beyond, champions the decision to delay childbearing, arguing that women who wait until they are ready for motherhood tend to be wealthier, more stable and satisfied in their careers and partnerships, and more emotionally mature. The author considers how adoption and reproductive technologies can offer older women (thirty-five years and up), singles, and lesbians the opportunity to become mothers when they are good and ready, after they have established themselves, sowed their wild oats, and had their adventures. My more diverse study participants agree with this notion of readiness up to a point. Consider this example from one of Gregory's interviews with a lawyer and single mother named Andrea, who adopted when she was forty-four years old:

You've gotten to travel, you've gotten to do stuff that's just for you, you've gotten to have the outrageous car, the outrageous handbag that cost too much money, take the most wonderful trips, not have to worry about getting a sitter. And so for me, at this point in time in my life, it's all good. . . . I'm happy, and I think that their happiness depends largely on your happiness. And if you aren't capable of taking care of yourself, and you aren't having a satisfying life, they are not having a satisfying life. And I think that in my twenties, I would have felt like I was missing something. (Gregory 2007, 260)

Andrea's veiled indictment of mothers less well off than she is and the symbolic cues that let others know she engages in higher-status modes of mothering underscore how class locations and other status disparities foster very different standards of readiness.

FINDING MR. RIGHT

The degree of focus on finding the right partner, which can be a rather diffuse goal, depends somewhat on age. The women in this study say that there is either still time or that the time has passed. Several of the single, heterosexual women wonder whether they should wait for the right man, or if they are older, they ponder the wisdom of having waited. Those whose primary romantic relationships are with women and those whose partners are men they deem unsuitable for fatherhood have dampened expectations of motherhood. And many of the women expend their energy examining their own emotional and material readiness to pair with a potential reproductive partner rather than actively seek someone to fit the position. Some of the women belong to communities that are more accepting of single motherhood (e.g., young African Americans, middle-class lesbians) and some to communities that are less accepting of this trend (e.g., middle-aged Latinas). For many of these reasons, the woman may find themselves torn:

> We didn't talk too much about the whole sperm donor thing, and that has been a big issue for me. Is it morally right to bring a child into this world who's going to only have a single parent? They'll always have those issues of "Who's my dad?" And it's kind of giving up the dream of Mr. Right and two and a half kids and the white picket fence. It's not a total nail in the coffin, but it certainly makes it more difficult to meet a man when you have a kid fathered by somebody else, even if that man is not in your life. —*Emily Reilly, thirty, white, single, fast food restaurant manager*

She wants to have children anyway, but she risks "giving up the [SNAF] dream" if she goes it alone. A woman can wait indefinitely for a partner, or she can enter motherhood, which may make her less attractive. For this reason many women delay making a decision, leaving events up to fate.

Many—but not all—of the women interviewed, including two of the lesbians (who, when partnered with men in their younger days, considered getting pregnant), focus on the need for an appropriate male partner with whom to have children. Marriage, most reason, implies that children are intended. The converse, singlehood, does not always mean that children are not part of the plan, but the status does complicate things considerably in instrumental, material, and ideological ways. Several of the interviewees tell of their frustration in not meeting eligible men in time to satisfy their biological clocks. Annie, for example, in commiserating with me over our shared childlessness, remarks that I am way ahead of her because at least I am married. This is a common outlook. As a case in point, Karen Tabb, a forty-nine-year-old teacher, expresses the idea that women should be married before considering having children. She has had several boyfriends but none were quite right for marriage and children, a fact she finds surprising, given her interest in children, but one she chooses not to dwell on. Her reason for not having children boils down to not having ever met the right man with whom to have them; this is why her childlessness just happened. Particularly the younger women, but also some of the older ones, insist that a man is unnecessary and that the lack of a partner will not prevent them from having children through adoption or a sperm bank, though most indicate that it would be nice to have a co-parent to share in the love and the responsibilities. Some of the women expected to have children with a particular partner, only to be disappointed to discover that he no longer wanted children or that he was not up to the task:

> We were all at the house and my nephew was two, I remember, and he wanted to play with my husband. My husband kind of shook him away. And I thought, "Oh no, that is not okay." In my heart, I was thinking, "Oh my God, how could you do that to a baby, to my nephew?" And I thought, "You want to have children?" Anyway it was wrong to me anyhow. . . . I mean I would just love to have a baby, but I'm not just going to go have a baby. I'm not just going to find somebody and be like, "You look nice; would you be the father of my child?" [*Laughs*] I mean it had to be real, it had to be a relationship that was going to last, like have a father and have a family, and what have you. —*Penny Ortiz, fifty-two, Latina, single, guidance counselor*

Penny remembers being "ready to have a baby" in her twenties. This readiness stemmed from feeling secure in her romantic relationship. But this particular boyfriend was not ready or not interested. Later, she sadly accepts that the man she married, despite his keen interest in having children, is not father material. Thus, she never becomes ready to have a child with him and never does have a baby. Many would look at Penny's life—noting her master's degree; career ambitions; her blithe, spur-of-the-moment travel expeditions; her frequent fun evenings out with friends—and dismiss her as another of those feminists who egocentrically indulges herself instead of settling down and becoming a mother as socially expected. As a society, we generally forget men's role in delayed childbearing, whether it is their reluctance to pursue having children or their failure to measure up as potential fathers. And certainly men's delayed parenthood is much less pathologized than that of women.

Gloria Owusu, in contrast to Penny, who stuck it out for a time, swiftly ditches her relationship when it becomes clear that the man does not want to have children with her. In my conversations with her, she sounds resigned to having children without a partner and expresses mild concern that her marketability will diminish should she adopt on her own. Unlike some women, Gloria feels ready even without the male partner. This divergence is partly the result of changing societal norms regarding the standard life course, as well as individual differences between women. Jessie Silva, whose husband seemed as though he would never be ready, broke off the relationship and later began a long-term partnership with a woman:

> It was always my journey. And I was thinking about it
> when I was married, too. It was something that I deep
> down always wanted so I was looking for a partner to
> have that with. Because I thought I had to do it with
> somebody else. I didn't think I could do it alone. That
> wasn't what I thought that I could do. So when I got into

my relationship with [her] I knew that our relationship wasn't going to go that way. And she wasn't ready. I just said, "This is what I'm doing. . . . I'm thirty-four and I'm going to adopt and it's going to take me a while and this is what I'm going to do." —*Jessie Silva, forty-two, white, queer, hair stylist*

As evident with Jessie's comments, having a partner is not solely about getting pregnant or about building a Standard North American Family. It is also about having another adult with whom to share the work of parenting and presumably to share the joys and intimacy. Several of the women for whom childlessness just happened never achieve sufficient readiness because they do not think they could do it alone. But Jessie evolves in her thinking, first believing that she needed to become pregnant with her husband, then that she merely needed a life partner to be ready for motherhood, and then finally recognizing that she can mother without either. Conservative initiatives, like George W. Bush's Marriage Initiative and anti–gay marriage bills notwithstanding, more and more families are female headed. This increase in acceptable family types allows women like Jessie to go against the grain with less stigma—and with a small measure of structural support. She receives some financial assistance, for example, from the state and federal governments for adopting a "special needs" (i.e., an ethnic minority, "drug-exposed") child.

Martina Klett-Davies's work (2007) on "lone motherhood" among welfare recipients in England and Germany develops several categories of single mothers: pioneers, copers, strugglers, and borderliners. Single motherhood is a feminist project for the pioneers, a temporary, improvable state for copers, an overwhelming trap for the strugglers, and a mix of these for the borderliners. It is important to note that state dependence does not preclude single motherhood from being an emancipatory experience. As Klett-Davies points out, it is easy to imagine a wealthy mother who stays in an unsatisfying marriage because of financial considerations as well as to imagine a poorer woman who feels the freedom of controlling her own meager spending. Klett-Davies's typology can be applied to childless and infertile women's predictions about their potential motherhood. There are those, like Jessie Silva, who declare their womanhood despite the "bodily disruption" of infertility and resolutely chart a course toward motherhood without a partner. More common among the study participants are those women who are reminiscent of the "copers."

Gloria Owusu and Emily Reilly, for example, were testing the waters of insemination and adoption—looking at the catalogs and getting certified as foster parents—when I met with them. Both worry somewhat about their chances of finding romantic partners after acquiring children, but they seem to think that as long as the possibility was there, they might just forge ahead into single motherhood. The prospective strugglers include women like Penny Ortiz, Karen Tabb, and Lourdes Garcia, all women in their fifties (or almost) for whom nonmotherhood "just happened," who doubt their ability to handle the financial and emotional demands of single motherhood. These women, raised before the second-wave women's movement of the 1970s, also allude to—in varying degrees—their concern about the legitimacy of children born out of wedlock and about the moral correctness of single motherhood. But the possibilities for women have changed in recent decades, concomitant with growing numbers of single mothers across the Western industrialized world (Duncan and Pfau-Effinger 2000). The youngest women in this study, the three African American women under twenty-six, predict single motherhood as a struggle if it were to happen right now. Nevertheless, provided they reach certain goals toward self-sufficiency, they welcome it.

The women in this study must parlay their own inclinations and choices about motherhood through the scrim of traditional notions of family and women's place in society. To say that women like Karen or Penny are "voluntarily" childless elides the fact that any choice they make is subject to social regulation. Women are expected to have children, and they are expected to get married. But these expectations are not an either/or proposition, nor are they mutually dependent. For women who want children, finding Mr. Right can be the only way out of this bind, a course wherein they can have children in comfortable, socially approved SNAF fashion. Those nervy singles and lesbians (who may also be medically infertile) who decide to make the effort to get pregnant and raise a child outside the institution of heterosexual marriage, make the decision to fulfill one mandate and forgo the other, but to do this they also have to decide *when* this is going to happen.

FINDING THE RIGHT TIME

> I just wasn't ready for it at that time. I wasn't ready for marriage either. I wasn't ready then to raise his kids and have more kids. I just wasn't ready for kids at that time. I mean, I loved picking up my nieces and nephews for the day; but I took them back afterwards. [Laughs] All my friends in high school had children before we graduated high school. I was the only one that did not have a child in high school. I seen what my sister went through being sixteen. Actually, [laughing] I didn't lose my virginity until I was out of high school because I was just so scared of being pregnant. And, I think about it now and I think, "God I should have done it" [laughs]; maybe I would have had more kids. I was just, kind of a little wild too, you know, being young. And, I wasn't ready to settle down. So my girlfriends in high school were having their

babies and dropping out, and I was into having fun and going out and partying and having a good time. —*Lupe Jimenez, forty-one, Latina, married, electronics technician*

The right time is, of course, an undefined objective, one influenced by others' opinions, by personal ambitions, by practical goals, and by age. As Lupe's comments show, laments about timing often occur in hindsight. She wishes she had had sex in high school (the search for Mr. Right be damned) because she may have had more children, and consequently she would now feel more successful as a mother and as a woman. In a reversal of popular narratives about teenage girls' wildness, Lupe sees her friends' pregnancies as an incentive for settling down, while she characterizes her own high school self as a partier who avoided pregnancy in favor of fun.

Readiness is not an exclusively personal experience or state of being. Many people in the lives of these women, especially their mothers, employers, friends, and partners, express their opinions about when they think the women are ready for motherhood. The women I spoke with note their mothers' warnings about their decreasing fertility over time, for example. They also bristle at—yet still mull over—other people's suggestions about timing:

> I can't believe she said that yesterday. I told [the director of the adoption agency] that I was between jobs and she was like, "Why don't you take the application back and, when you get a job, come back." I am like, "Take my application now before I change my mind." I should have something going on. . . . So you know, keep it. I don't want to take it back. I been meditating about this. I been thinking about—I been setting my mind to this and I'm *ready*. —*LaWanda Jackson, forty-two, African American, single, nursing assistant*

Most of my friends have children already. And many of them had them young—eighteen, nineteen, twenty. And everybody says, "Annie, you should have a child." And I'm like, "I'm not ready to have a child." This is what I thought. I mean, sometimes I think, what will I do with a child? I can barely take care of myself. And then sometimes I feel like maybe having a child would help me direct my purpose in life, try to focus my efforts on something specific. —*Annie Adoyo, thirty, second-generation African immigrant, single, student*

All the people would say, "It's time. Your clock is ticking." It's like society says, my coworkers said, "You should start having children now." I'm like, "Leave me alone." See, society is expecting me to have children at a certain age. Now I'm close to thirty-five and I'm not having any children and some other professional will tell me, "Hey, you should start having children because the older you get the more difficult it gets." —*Serena Lopez, thirty-nine, Latina, married, pharmacy technician*

Despite the fact that LaWanda feels ready, the adoption director, an outsider, tells her she cannot become a mother at this time, at least not through that avenue. Her prospects for motherhood are beholden to a bureaucrat's assessment of her readiness. Readiness is not the personal choice Gregory (2007) and others make it out to be. Annie is told that she is ready when she thinks she is not. She equivocates on this, seeming to take her friends' remarks under advisement. She may not be financially stable—or, in her particular case, as healthy as she ideally could be—but Annie thinks that having a child might help her to embrace her adult responsibilities. She is ready for motherhood for the same reason that some young adults enter the military—to be forced to grow up. In fact, several of the women make this claim that motherhood "makes a woman out of you."

Other women feel they must meet a number of personal and professional goals (hypothetically) *before* having children:

> I want a daughter, I really do. But I don't want a baby now. . . . I don't have the finances to be able to take care of a baby. And when I do have her, I want to be able to spoil her. You hear a lot of people say that. And I don't just mean financially. I want to be at her school when she has a field trip. Of course I want her to be well taken care of. I just want to be as *ready* as possible. I want to have a baby. Not in the near, near, near future, but after I've gotten a degree. After I'm settled into what Nicole wants to do. Which is be a mortician . . . after I'm established, around twenty-six, twenty-seven. But once I get there, I don't want to be old. I want to enjoy her childhood.
> —*Nicole Lambert, twenty, African American, single, student*

Media stories, pundits, and common stereotypes promote the idea that delayed childbearing is selfish. These women argue just the opposite, that delayed childbearing is more *selfless* and responsible. The women point out that they need time to do what they want to do, including getting an education, establishing a satisfying career, and, for the one who can afford it, having adventures (like Jennifer West, the forty-six-year-old engineer who surfed in many countries). For thirty-nine-year-old Serena Lopez, the goal is to solidify her new marriage and buy a house in preparation for children. Motherhood, as a life stage, necessitates clearing the calendar, as it were, because, as Nicole indicates, they wish to "spoil" their future children. Because they anticipate conforming to an intensive mothering ideal (Hays

1998) and because they need to earn a living, some delay child-bearing past their most fertile years.

Women must constantly negotiate a suite of new choices, but compared to the traditional ideal, their decisions often make them feel as if they are coming up short. Jennifer, for example, feels that she lost the opportunity to birth a child because she simply waited too long, always thinking that there was still time. She stands out as one of the few participants in this project who approximate the careerist stereotype—that woman who (ill advisedly) pursues the glory of a high-powered career and then is (stupidly) crestfallen when she finally decides too late to pursue motherhood. This allegory, shot through with schadenfreude at women who apparently do not know their place, or alternatively, at snobby women who cannot appreciate their privileges, does not resonate with most of my interview population. They are hardworking and goal-oriented (but not particularly career-track) professionals: most have working-class occupations and modest lifestyles, and they must work to live (not that they do not enjoy their work). The tired discourse that modern women are to blame because they sacrifice their fertility for their careers may lack explanatory power, but it still weighs on the consciences of infertile and childless women.

Some women offer the perspective that having a child is one of their goals in life, something else to strive for:

> I think that, for me, that's on my list of things to do in my life is have a baby. I feel like there's this emphasis on experiences in society, and that's one experience I want to have, being pregnant. —*Emily Reilly, thirty, white, single, fast food manager*

> I've never seen children and yearned, "I want my own." I just enjoyed seeing them. But I have not got to the

point where I see a child and think, "I wish that was me," no. But I think just society, and because of all the people I know, I'm the last one who hasn't married and had kids, so I think about that, but I've not been one to follow the crowd and keep up with the Joneses anyway. I just think for me, personally, it's time to make that initial step [toward having children].

—*Gloria Owusu, thirty-eight, African American, single, project manager*

Emily later tells me that riding a motorcycle is also on that list. Her concept of having a baby is, in part, checking off an item on life's to-do list. Gloria, too, does not "yearn" for a child, does not come off as at all forlorn, but instead matter-of-factly recognizes that she has reached a predetermined time for becoming a mother, something she is especially ready for now that her younger brother has moved out, leaving her with nobody to nurture. Both women are single and both desire pregnancy but, in keeping with their purposefulness, have another option—adoption—lined up as well. Emily and Gloria differ from the Infertile Woman supposedly preoccupied with the need to conceive in that they talk casually, almost flippantly at times, of having children as something they plan to do alongside all their other pursuits. Maybe this attitude stems from a psychological defense mechanism in which they do not want to come off as wanting a child too much, or perhaps they do not wish to test fate. Even if true, that is not the whole story. Ticking off motherhood from a list is not just a metaphor for instrumental consumerism but an acknowledgment and anticipation of motherhood as a *process* that engenders existential human connection. They want the life-enriching experience, but that aspiration does not define them.

AGE TALK

The women I talked with contend that a woman can be too young or too old to become a mother. However, they differ drastically in their views of what age range is appropriate. Several, especially the poorer, younger African American women and the Latinas I interviewed, suggest the early to mid-twenties as the best age for having children. Robin Smith, a fertility worker, marvels at the youth of the few women of color who come to her clinic for insemination; they tend to be around age twenty-five, she says, already worrying about aging out of their prime. Her usual clients are white and well beyond their mid-thirties, many into their late forties. The older African American women and all of the white women say that thirty is the perfect age to begin having children. By that time, they loosely imply, women should be settled in terms of relationships, financial stability, and their career paths. Since their standpoints vary by race and age, it makes sense to examine the national birth rates of these cohorts. The American Community Survey (US Census Bureau 2008) provides the statistics in Table 1.

TABLE 1.

Births per 1,000 in the last 12 months by age and race
(US Census Bureau 2008)

	15–19	20–24	25–29	30–34	35–39	40–44
White	16.7	48.6	42.5	29.7	11.4	2.5
Black	30.1	53.1	30.6	17.2	2.9	0
Hispanic	45.6	59.5	31.4	30	6.6	6
Asian	10.3	16.3	43.3	33.9	31.2	0

In comparison to black women and white women, Asian women have exceptionally low birthrates overall, and Hispanic women have particularly high ones. Looking more closely at the age at first birth between black women and white women, though, it becomes evident that fewer and fewer black women have their first child as they approach thirty and beyond. Interestingly, the highest current fertility (i.e., not cumulative numbers of children) by any category studied (e.g., income, educational attainment, race, age) occurred among women with graduate or professional degrees who had sixty-seven births per one thousand!

These patterns have several implications for childless and infertile women. First, because they wait to find a partner and/or achieve stability, they tend to get serious about birthing (or adopting) a child much later than their peers, who have children more easily without as much forethought. Second, that black teenagers have twice as many births as white teenagers bears out in the experience of the young African American women in this study who feel like social oddities—expressing to me their pride and autonomy as well as their defensiveness and a little consternation—as nonmothers at the youthful ages of nineteen, twenty, and twenty-five. Third, the fact that highly educated women were the most likely to become mothers in 2006 speaks to the social milieu in which women routinely control their reproduction with birth control, abortion, and the intentional timing of "conception" and in which many make decisions to enter motherhood only after completing their education. It is not just that women are having children later—women always have had children into their forties—it is that some are having children for the first time later in life. The ideal life course for women, particularly in terms of entering motherhood, is changing; and medical interventions, or simply knowing that they are available if needed, enters into the decision making. Just like other American women, many infertile and childless women spend their years between puberty and menopause avoiding pregnancy or pursuing pregnancy, contingent in part on their proximity to a small—but moveable—age window. Race and class background likely influence the age parameters, and as individual women age, some—but certainly not all—adjust upward their notion of the ideal time to become mothers.

The medical and census-taking definition of childbearing age is fifteen to forty-four, though of course there are plenty of exceptions. The more restrictive social definitions to which the women I interviewed refer involve a mainstream disdain for teenage motherhood and a vague aversion to pregnancy among women over thirty-five. Beginning at age thirty-five, women who become pregnant are almost universally labeled "high risk" (see Simonds et al. 2007) and pressured to submit to umpteen invasive diagnostic tests (Rapp 1999). Even at age thirty—or even twenty-five, as interviewee Azra Alic laments—women who visit infertility clinics not only begin to hear about their decreasing chances of a "healthy" or "successful" pregnancy but also get slapped with incrementally higher fees with each birthday. Accordingly, age constrains women's ability to accomplish readiness for childbearing (and childrearing more generally). The question for women becomes: can I satisfy other aspects of readiness like finding a suitable partner, becoming financially stable, and preparing myself emotionally and psychologically in time to get pregnant—or to adopt before I am too old for childrearing? This question is at the forefront of some of their minds, but for others it remains abstract. Consider the passages below, which roughly correspond to chronological life-course stages as they relate to motherhood:

> I can still have kids but it can take a long time and I don't have that much time. I'm thirty now so it's five years since my first surgery. I don't want to be forty and still—you

know what I mean? So they are suggesting IVF. —*Azra Alic, thirty, Bosnian immigrant, engaged, apartment manager*

When I was twenty-six, nothing was happening, no relationships to speak of, I had said that when I am thirty-five, if I am not married, I will have my own by whatever means. —*Gloria Owusu, thirty-eight, African American, single, project manager*

So I went to my gynecologist, who said that there was a pretty slim chance of my getting pregnant, because by the time I went, I think I was in my late thirties, maybe thirty-seven or thirty-eight. And so I went and my gynecologist said, "It's not looking too great" . . . so they did all these tests, and my uterus was loaded with fibroids. —*Dianne Jacobsen, fifty-six, white, single, life coach*

We did try. We tried a lot more times. To this day, my mom will still tell me to try again. I'm going to be forty-two years old. [*Laughs*] I'm done! —*Lupe Jimenez, forty-one, Latina, married, electronics technician*

You see all the excitement of a new baby and all that. But it doesn't give me any ideas of wanting to be in her place. [*Laughs*] Besides that, I'm past my time, you know. —*Iris Hernandez, fifty-four, Latina, office assistant*

Some of these women hear the proverbial biological clock ticking, and others are too busy to listen; but all relate their awareness of the impact of time and age on their fertility/infertility or status as mothers/nonmothers. Nicole, quoted further above, has no reason to doubt her fertility, and she envisions her late twenties as the best age to enter motherhood. Azra, a few years older and already encountering problems with her reproductive system, worries about time as she accelerates her involvement with medically assisted conception. Beginning at age twenty-five, she tries surgery, then a hysterosalpingogram (HSG) to examine and clear her fallopian tubes. She takes Clomid to help her ovulate and then tries injectable fertility drugs before starting IVF. She relates a sense of urgency now, owing to fears that she may not be able to get pregnant and carry to term. Azra insists on waiting to marry her fiancé until she can prove her fertility. She explains that she does not want to "waste his time" or limit his opportunity for fatherhood, something she says he does not even realize may eventually become more important to him than she is. She is doubly unhappy about her infertility because, to her, it *may* (she is not consistent about this) also spell the end of her relationship—and her identity as a woman. Gloria, as noted earlier, plans for the contingency that she will not find the right partner in time and sets an age by which time she will make a withdrawal from the sperm bank or adopt a child (domestically). By contrast, Karen Tabb reports having been untroubled when she was approaching thirty, even though her mother warned her that time was running out. She, like many others I interviewed, thought there would be time later on to pursue motherhood. For Dianne time ran out early. Her mother reminded her that menopause tends to start early in her family, but Dianne was still caught unawares, discovering that her body would not cooperate once she was ready to get pregnant. Lupe attempted to have a second child and experienced only debilitating miscarriages. She has let go of any hope or intention to have more, but her mother still thinks that Lupe has time left in which to try for another. (Mothers' advice is a leitmotif in these interviews, and it is nearly always about advising daughters on their readiness for motherhood. For their part the daughters often deliberately exclude their judgmental, worrying, or confused mothers from full knowledge of their goals surrounding motherhood or childfree living.) Finally, Iris, chuckling at the seemingly ridiculous idea that she would still want to become a mother, reminds me that she is "past [her] time," that she is on the other side of menopause and no longer interested in pregnancy or adoption.

These snippets from several infertile and childless women's lives highlight the theme of time that shadows women's childbearing years and beyond. Sociologist Elisabeth Ettore (2002) describes reproduction as a structured social practice that covers a wide expanse of time and space. Thinking about motherhood probably begins for most women in girlhood as they see their own mothers at work and as they play house and play with dolls, rehearsing their presumed destiny. It does not end at the age of forty-four, whether or not women have had children. And assumptions about motherhood and nonmotherhood impact women's lives in many environments: within families, at work, among friends, in interactions with strangers. But the actual span of time when a woman can enter motherhood is rather small if one takes into account the myriad personal, biological, and social cues for readiness that must first appear.

A vague sense that there must still be time—when indeed there was not—influenced the childlessness or age-related infertility, or secondary infertility of many:

> I say well, I still want to have a child. There are women in their forties having [babies]—like my sister-in-law when she was thirty-nine. The day before her fortieth birthday she had my niece, and her sister tried for like six months and she was forty-one, and had a healthy boy. So you hear stories about Holly Hunter, how she had twins, and she's forty-seven. —*Talia Stein, forty-one, white, single, home healthcare aide*

Knowledge of celebrities giving birth later in life persuades some women that this practice is the new norm, even desirable, or at least is relatively free of negative consequences. They all know about the miracles of assisted conception and the attendant technologies, something few of them pursue. Nullifying a hypothesis of mine, these women do not seem to experience a sense of relative deprivation; many do not mention the cost prohibitions; they do not decry the policies that discourage singles and lesbians from accessing services; they do not point out that surrogacy arrangements might be difficult to find and arrange for women of color or for working-class women; and they do not seem to feel left out of that scene at all. If they want or wanted to become mothers badly enough, they suggest, they will find or would have found their way through the medical or adoption bureaucracies (about which many know relatively little), or they would informally adopt a relative's child (two mentioned this solution). Instead, they indicate that they are insufficiently motivated. Greil et al. (2009) name motivation to become mothers as one of the factors behind seeking help with infertility. What motivates women to plow through the thickets of ART and adoption bureaucracies? Material and ideological barriers aside, and time constraints notwithstanding, the women I talked with avoid coming to any decisions about motherhood. Some point to examples within their own families: of aunts, older sisters, mothers, and grandmothers who gave birth into their forties. Several take a pragmatic view of their childlessness, choosing to extol the many benefits of childfree living but not giving those benefits as the *reason* for their childlessness.

With all these possibilities in the backs of their minds, it is easy to ignore the creeping passage of time. Their experiences are at odds with those of Robin Smith's infertility patients (in a nod to the consumerist conception of infertile women, she calls them "clients"). They race against time, ratcheting up their treatments, increasing frequency, degree of invasiveness, and levels of medical expertise as they age, all in pursuit of pregnancy before it is too late. This description conflates the medical definition of infertility with the actions of the infertility clients. The reason many of the respondents differ from these "infertile" women may simply be because they avoided, limited, or delayed medicalization, whether intentionally or not, and remained focused on more pressing aspects of their lives.

It is a well-worn criticism of contemporary society that women must somehow complete their education and mount fulfilling, self-supporting careers while also fitting in pregnancy, childbirth, and childrearing. Virtually all the women I spoke with—women who are either childless, infertile, or both—constantly mention the virtuous real moms who mother with all they have. Their own childless or infertile status partially results from an acceptance of this unattainable ideal. They await readiness for motherhood, sometimes indefinitely as they hope to find the right partner, to achieve their other goals, to encounter the right time, and to reach—but not pass—the prime age. As a society we expect women to work out these problems on their own (and, to a lesser degree, with their partners), instead of calling on society to support mothers or even calling into question individualistic cultural models that shun communal living and adopt isolating, neolocal residence patterns. The existing system promotes infertility and childlessness by not supporting women's childbearing earlier in their lives, effectively shutting some women out of motherhood. The deferment of any explicit planning of many of these women's life courses (and perhaps this kind of planning is a yuppie construction just as infertility is often seen as a yuppie disease) stems from the complexity involved in attaining readiness for motherhood and a steadfast belief that motherhood is not wholly an achievement; rather, it is somewhat mystical—that is, ascribed by unseen forces.

5

ASCRIBED MOTHERHOOD

Instead of blaming society or personal failure, the women I talked with, who tend to find their infertility or childlessness to be mostly a positive or neutral outcome, commonly attribute their condition to chance or "God's will" or "God's plan" for them. They overwhelmingly attribute the occurrence of motherhood or nonmotherhood to forces beyond their control, supernatural influences that may or may not be affected by women's behavior. More than two-thirds of them brought up the supernatural in accounting for their infertility and/or childlessness, not merely as a coping mechanism but as a driving force. Motherhood to them is primarily an ascribed role, not an achieved one. This view emerges as the exact opposite of the (exaggerated) pursuit by the Infertile Woman to get pregnant even if it means submitting to dangerous, improbable, morally questionable, or intrusive treatments. The multi-billion-dollar-per-year financial interest in women's pursuit of motherhood at all costs benefits from a focus on achieving motherhood. It places the power in the hands of unfeeling technogods who perform the medical miracles instead of— from the perspective of many of the women in this study—in God's loving hands (or, for some of the women, the benevolent, omniscient, animistic "universe"):

I mean I'm sure if God put [a baby] in my life, I'd do it, but what I think of the choice, I think God has made me an auntie for a reason. I say that repeatedly. . . . I never really know what the plan is because He's got it, but the plan was: you're an auntie because you got plenty to do with all your nieces and nephews and friends' babies. . . . So I think I just accepted the fact that God did not want to bless me with children but bless me as an auntie and then move on. —*Penny Ortiz, fifty-two, Latina, single, guidance counselor*

Penny accepts her childlessness with the comforting realization that there is a greater plan than any one she could have predicted or designed herself. It is not enough for her to say that she was preoccupied with other satisfying life pursuits: the dominant discourse does not sufficiently legitimate that path to fulfillment for women. She was meant to be the one free to provide additional support to others' children (and, as she details later, to care for her elderly parents). In this way of thinking, some women attempt to manipulate the grand design, sometimes concluding that individuals do not hold that kind of power:

> They all knew we were trying to get pregnant; they were rooting for us. And the whole time I felt like so restless; I wanted to get pregnant so bad while we were down there and I remember when we left, one of the boys said to us [*whispers*], "I just know next time we see you, you're going to have a little brown fuzzy headed little girl." Like I almost started crying the way he said it. And then it's so weird because I came back and I was so restless. I went through the IUI, it was like I was trying everything in my powers that I knew how to do because I wasn't

really ready to take that step for IVF. And I was doing everything I could. I took that next step further on the fost-adopt and even the next step further on to adoption. And the whole time—I started thinking about it after we got [our adopted daughter]—that's when she was conceived . . . while we were down there in Costa Rica. So it was like the whole time I was just so restless, maybe I knew my baby was coming. —*Jennifer West, forty-six, Latina, married, engineer*

God really does have a plan because now I can look back and go, "Ohh. This is what He was doing. Hey, good planning, God!" It would've been nice if He would've warned me. But I just think it's God's plan. And He knows when you're ready for it and when you're not and if you should, if you can't. I think of one of my girlfriends from high school who wanted—she had her daughter— and she wanted another baby so bad and she had so many miscarriages and she finally had her baby. And he was born with this very, very rare disease and I can't remember what they call it, but the little guy had so many things wrong with him. And she would forever have to take care of that little guy. I mean, I don't know how long they live, supposedly they don't live very long . . . and often I thought that she wanted so badly to have this baby and she finally got to have him but it wasn't God's plan. He didn't want her to have a baby." —*Penny Ortiz, fifty-two, Latina, single, guidance counselor*

Jennifer recalls a child's prophecy and her own eerie restlessness, indications of the supernatural at work. She was just passing the time by trying some low-tech assisted conception methods and taking incremental steps toward adoption (a process she did not even complete until after the placement); meanwhile, her adopted daughter-to-be had already been conceived and was ostensibly waiting to become Jennifer's baby. From the vantage point of happy motherhood, she is able to look back and (re)construct events as proof that her infertility, her unsuccessful attempts at pregnancy, and her eventual adoption were preordained by an all-knowing force, one she unconsciously detected as evident in her otherwise unexplained restlessness. She does not report desperation or frustration so much as a state of flux. Unlike Penny, Jennifer is not overtly religious. But assigning power to another plane elevates her experience, something she may need as evidenced by the unflattering way she describes fertility clinics and the adoption bureaucracy. Instead of being a path that must be metaphorically bushwhacked and endured, her journey's twists and turns provide opportunity for self-realization and inspiration. Penny's God has more complex motivations. You have to be careful what you wish for. Trying too hard to circumvent His will, His eternal plan, instead of accepting—even embracing—your fate as Penny does can result in devastating consequences. The woman in Penny's story who could not accept her secondary infertility finally got the baby she wanted "so bad[ly]" . . . along with a large, punitive dose of heartbreak.

Magical Motherhood

For others, letting go of control, putting one's faith in God's plan, or drawing on magical forces is the most likely route to motherhood (or, at the very least, it cannot hurt):

> You want to hear a miracle? One of our friends in church, her husband was trying to have a baby for five years. And I just talked to her and told her that God and Jesus said that whatever you ask in his name, you shall

receive. Once you have faith. I prayed over her and I said to her, "Raise your hands to the Lord Jesus and say, 'Thank you, Lord Jesus, for giving me my baby right now.'" The faith in things we haven't seen yet. A few months later she got pregnant. She has a little girl now. Her name is Aakalijah. She's five months. —*LaWanda Jackson, forty-two, African American, single, nursing assistant*

If you focus on your intent and eliminate the word "want," let that go, but visualize you being pregnant, being a mother, it'll manifest itself. —*Talia Stein, forty-one, white, single, home healthcare aide*

LaWanda, an evangelical, encourages an acquaintance's faith, and the woman gets pregnant. For some women, trust in fate or in God must precede the fulfillment of wishes. The ubiquitous —and, frankly, irritating—advice to women trying to get pregnant to "just relax" is a homologous assumption from the secular world. Both ideas subtly blame women for their own infertility and scorn desperation. Harking back to Puritan ideology, wanting something too much leads to curses and jinxes since people have failed to have enough faith. By contrast, Robin Smith, a forty-two-year-old partnered lesbian, uses the supernatural casually, treating it as yet another possibly helpful option among so many, saying in reference to her clients' interest in her fertility journey, "I'm not real picky about which energy it is we're tapping into. We'll take whatever you've got." Her clinic promotes the use of a dizzying array of herbs and tonics, diets, acupuncture, massage, yoga, and meditation along with more prosaic correctives like fertility drugs, HSGs, and other medical procedures. She points out that acupuncture, massage, yoga, and meditation help clients relax to improve fertilization odds (again the old warning that blames women), relax to get through invasive and taxing process of fertility treatment (again and again), and to harness supernatural energies. Another, more latent function may be to deflect responsibility for the effectiveness of treatment by hinting that success or failure is ultimately up to the supernatural, not to the individual doctors and fertility clinics.

Magic can also stand in for "holism" in the notoriously alienating world of fertility treatment. At one clinic I witnessed routinized summoning of supernatural powers. After a brief IUI procedure in which the (tardy) doctor barely glanced at me before inserting the syringe (and allowing my partner to perform the symbolic and practical act of "pushing the plunger"), the counselor in an equally indifferent manner then grabbed two rattles she described as "fertility idols" and shook them over my body for "good luck." We tolerated this ritual fourteen times for seven unsuccessful cycles.

For several of the women I spoke with, the supernatural is more meaningful and allows control to shift away from doctors and other authorities in ways that are liberating for women. It is a common feeling among adoptive parents that their child is exactly the right one for them, a feeling attributed here to having met in a past life. Jessie Silva tells me that once she "let go" of any residual anger at her medical encounters, at the frustrating adoption process, and at the unfairness of her infertility, and "opened her heart," her daughter's soul preternaturally perceived this and became willing to come into her life. Had I interviewed her—or any of the other women—before they made peace with their situations, I may have reached very different conclusions. But based on the narrative I heard, women like Jessie place the bulk of their faith in higher powers instead of with medical and adoption-system authorities. She says she never feared losing her daughter (whom she first fostered) to birth-family reunification because, even though the social workers tried to "scare" her, she tapped into her own spirituality and "just *knew*" that she and the child "belonged together."

Loss of control is one of the most often cited negative impacts of assisted conception (Becker 2000). Women like Jessie, while taking back some of this control herself ("opening her heart") and giving a significant measure of control over to the universe, symbolically wrest it away from those same doctors who are told by advertisers that "you are their only hope." Nicole's comments assert this view:

> If I experience something like the doctor telling me I won't ever be able to have a baby, I'll take that and throw it out the window. Honestly. Just because of past situations and the people they've seen? Maybe God is saying, "Now is not the time for you to have a baby." But that's not to say that you won't ever be able to. I believe that if it's in His will for me to have a child, then I don't care what the doctor says. I don't care how many degrees they have. If it's in God's will for me, then I will have a child, but in His time. . . . My prayer wouldn't be, "Oh God, give me a baby." Honestly. It would be, "Okay, I see it's not happening now in your time" . . . once you realize that you don't have control over things you say, "Okay, well it's out of my hands. I've tried everything there is."

Kristin Wilson: What would you try?

> As far as having a baby, adoption is always an option. But if that's not what I want to do, I wouldn't do that. I could take in a relative, but you usually want to have your own. But once you see that the only thing bringing fulfillment is being able to carry a baby that you and someone else created, once you see that that's not happening, you say,

"Okay, I'm going to hold off. And basically leave it in God's hands." —*Nicole Lambert, twenty, African American, single, student*

Nicole's rhetoric does not always stay consistent, but her position that God knows more than doctors do reverberates throughout this collection of interviews. Relinquishing control to God is preferable to giving over to doctors. This attitude should be read neither as overly traditional nor as psychological self-protection. Ironically, it is a way for women to own their life trajectories despite the vicissitudes of their bodies and their life opportunities.

Some of the women—instead of waiting patiently for God's blessing or calling on the supernatural to hurry up and make them mothers (as Robin does)—indicate that God called or may call them. LaWanda Jackson, a forty-two-year-old nurse's aide, for example, decides to look into adoption when she keeps hearing mention of it, encountering messages that she interprets as being hailed directly by God to do her duty and take in a needy child. She thinks she is now really ready, particularly because she is lonely, and she longs for the companionship and an opportunity to create the kind of special mother-daughter bond she never experienced with her own mother. Like many of the women who feel called to motherhood, she knows that she will be a good mother; and God apparently knows that, too, and will soon bless her with a child.

Holy Paternalism
The colonial concept of "blessing" turns up frequently in women's discussions about having children. One is blessed or not blessed by God with children (also known as "blessings"). God blesses those who are ready to become mothers, whether they recognize their readiness or not, and does not bless those who

are neither ready nor deserving, whether or not they know why. Like the conventional model father, kind and benevolent, yet quick to mete out stern discipline when necessary, so goes the supernatural influence on motherhood:

> But the way it is right now, I am blessed I do not have kids. Because the situation, I see children are suffering so much. —*Lourdes Garcia, fifty-six, Latina, single, office assistant*

> I would consider adoption, but I would first want to experience pregnancy and everything like that. But I can say, it's a blessing. And you don't have visuals, a camcorder, but this mole on my hand, my mother has the same mole! The exact same mole in the exact same place. You can ask her if you don't believe me. It is such a miracle. It's like, what are the chances of me having this and my mother having the exact same mole and she adopted me? None of her other children have it. So we say that this is our mark from God, who says, "Nicole, this is your mother. This is your child." I don't think anything happens by chance. I believe God has allowed a time or preordained a time. And so I believe this was meant to happen. So yeah, my mother was of an age [forty-eight] when she adopted me. —*Nicole Lambert, twenty, African American, single, student*

> I said, "What bad luck we have." I tried this, it did not work. I tried this, it did not work. And sometimes I believe, it's spiritual too, some kind of power that did not want me to have any kids. So I said what I think is I'd rather live like this. I don't want. If I bring somebody to my life [i.e, adopt], maybe something—I get scared that

something will happen to that kid or something like that.
—*Zara Senai, forty-five, African immigrant, married, laboratory technician*

Nineteen-year-old Jamilah Washington points out that she is not yet blessed because God knows she is not ready, while Lourdes, too, is relieved to be blessed to not have children, as she feels incapable in the midst of a decaying society. Nicole recognizes that her mother adopted her right on time, according to God's plan. But others, like one of Robin Smith's clients and Zara, are not blessed; they are cursed. Robin's client and, certainly other women as well, may feel punished with infertility because they had abortions when they thought they were not ready to become mothers but when in fact God intended it. Karey Harwood (2007) wonders if undergoing ART is not an ascetic expression or absolution for known or unknown past sins; they brought their infertility on themselves and must suffer to undo it. The daily injections are modern-day flagellations (and, because of hot flashes, Clomid makes an apt hair shirt).

Nicole comments at one point, "God wouldn't give me anything I can't handle," referring to any accidental pregnancies—and children—she might have (she claims at times that she doesn't believe in abortion, though she vacillates on this issue). Zara, like many others, wonders what she did to deserve such bad luck. In the quotation above, Zara talks about her fear that the curse may be contagious to those who are close to her. She suffered the pain of many fibroids in her uterus—an organ she refuses to have removed from her body, believing it to be the essence of her womanhood—and unwittingly doomed her husband to worrying about her health and to fatherlessness. At his behest, they attempted to adopt a little boy, a boy they received a photograph of prior to the adoption; but, sadly, the boy died of pneumonia before they met him. After this emotional blow, she decided that she better not try to become a mother against the will of some spiritual power lest she transfer her curse to other potential children. For her, this spiritual power is dangerous and maybe not benevolent at all.

Yet women do sometimes turn to the supernatural to help them cope with infertility or childlessness. The relatively worse condition of a coworker's daughter, who is unable to bear children at all because of a malformed uterus, helps Lupe, despite her own secondary infertility, feel grateful that she already had a son. She, like a few others, credits a single, fated moment in which she "snapped out of it" and into this enlightenment. Hannah, the most irreligious of all the respondents, says that she does not believe in the occult but still allowed a medium to do some "feeling work" with her after her infertility diagnosis. Although the channeling does not bring a specific message, the psychic claims that an ancestor was attempting to contact her. Consulting with her mother, they decide that it must be a maiden aunt from Hungary who never had any children. Despite the fact that she denies believing in the supernatural aspects of this encounter, Hannah reflects on that aunt's life and commitment to progressive political work, finding it a helpful inspiration as she works to accept her infertility.

Chance

Chance signifies probability (as in odds), opportunity, and happenstance. Chalking up life's events to chance can be a more secular way of diffusing the power that influences who becomes a mother and when, and who does not or cannot. This concept regularly surfaces in the interviews:

> [The doctor] said I might have a chance to still get a tubal pregnancy so you know the opportunity still be there but the hole—there is still a little hole. Plus that

was back then; they didn't have all this high-tech stuff they have today. But I just lay there and boom. But yeah, so I tried then and I am like, okay, there's some hope; you can still have a chance to have a baby. But then it was like when I was trying, it didn't happen. —*LaWanda Jackson, forty-two, African American, single, nursing assistant*

And finally he said, "I think we have to remove those fibroids." It's like about nine of them now. And they said, "Okay, you have a fifty-fifty chance that maybe you will get pregnant, maybe you'll get scars. It's going to be hard. —*Zara Senai, forty-five, African immigrant, married, laboratory technician*

You pay for [ART] and stick yourself with needles all the time. For that baby, you're taking chances. It's like playing Russian roulette. —*LaWanda Jackson, forty-two, African American, single, nursing assistant*

I started going to church more often, trying to get involved in all the things. But at the same time like, "God, this divorce happened when I'm old and maybe I'll never get married again, maybe I'll never—last chance to have children." Right, I'm not going to go meet a guy and get pregnant right away. So last chance to have children. —*Serena Lopez, thirty-nine, Latina, married, pharmacy technician*

In LaWanda's first comment excerpted above, she uses the word "chance" twice: once to mean that she might have another ectopic pregnancy (therefore she feels that she should think twice before getting pregnant again) and once to mean that there is still a possibility that she may yet birth a baby (therefore she refuses to give up hope of finding another husband with whom to start a family). She explains that since she is aware that there is a medically defined chance, she can now leave it up to God to decide whether to bless her with a successful pregnancy. In the second excerpt, LaWanda shares her dubious view of ART, suggesting that women who do it are taking unwise risks, that they are endangering their health to get a baby. For women like Zara, doctors' use of "chance(s)" equates to calling the odds on their fertility potential. In many cases they stop short of trying every treatment available to them mainly because they believe their chances of success to be so small. Following fibroid surgery, Dianne has a "little window of opportunity" in which she could get pregnant before getting more fibroids and/or reaching menopause. She does not want to take the drugs involved. Some women—perhaps more set on biological motherhood and/or perhaps more accepting of anecdotal success stories— probably help keep the fertility industry afloat and further encourage more experimentation in reproductive medicine.

Zara reports being given a "fifty-fifty" chance to "maybe get pregnant." The meanings of these kinds of odds are obscured by their prevalent, inconsistent, colloquial, and incorrect use and by patient misunderstanding. Rayna Rapp (1999) notes similar problems with doctor-patient statistical discussions around prenatal test results. Statistical probabilities inform the recommendations of fertility doctors and the relative costs of treatment.

Biologists characterize human reproduction as inefficient and influenced by innumerable behavioral factors, including timing of intercourse, penis withdrawal patterns, washing, and environmental conditions (e.g., Tingen et al. 2004). The idea that there is a 20 to 30 percent chance of pregnancy in any given "exposure" during sex appears to be accepted dogma. My experience with infertility specialists reveals additional insight into the numbers game in the fertility world where statistical confusion reigns. The fertility specialists whom I saw in Atlanta did not provide any numbers. Instead they said that "most women" get pregnant within six cycles of IUI and "almost all" get pregnant within twelve. In California my doctor told me that I had a 3 to 5 percent chance of getting pregnant with each attempt at ICI (intracervical insemination) done at home and "double that" chance with IUI (intrauterine insemination) in his office. I wrote his statistics down and scoured the medical literature for some reference to back it up. I had no luck. Incidentally, I got pregnant twice, both times with the at-home ICI. He referred me to an IVF clinic after the first miscarriage, telling me that I would "probably" get pregnant "right away." The origin of the probabilities given to the few women I talked with who did interface with some medical intervention and to me is mysterious and probably arbitrary, the rough guess of a doctor. "Chance," when used by doctors, signifies not just scientific probability but also the relative amount of hope remaining. When there is a chance, there is hope. The quantifiable concept of chance transubstantiates into the metaphysical concept of hope. Miracles can happen, they might happen, and one must put one's faith in God's will, luck, medical miracles, or a combination of all three. Hannah is given excellent odds for getting pregnant with IVF, but she is not willing to take that bet:

> We started looking at IVF and you know, with my case, what I was quoted in terms of the chances of getting pregnant didn't sound good enough to me—

> Kristin Wilson: Do you know what they are?

> They were probably relatively high, I think 25 percent. But given our limited resources, they didn't seem good enough to put all of our money there. And with me it would have been pretty complicated. —*Hannah Johanson, thirty-nine, white, queer, married, teacher*

Though Hannah's quoted chances were as high as nature is supposed to be, she cannot leave her opportunity for motherhood up to chance. She expresses concern at the complexity involved, but she also refuses to put her faith (and her money) into a process that is not guaranteed. Adoption, she decides, is a better use of funds because the chances of a take-home baby are much higher, a choice many adoptive mothers make (see Jacobson 2008).

Penny Ortiz likens chance to serendipity. Her childlessness gives her the chance to fill an important niche, that of a godmother auntie and caretaker. This usage is consistent with her belief in God's master plan. This meaning underscores the belief by many of the women that motherhood is ascribed in spite of dominant narratives that emphasize it as an achievement (Ginsburg 1989). For Penny this concept of "chance" allows her a positive spin on childlessness. It is opportunity knocking at the door.

Mary Benson says, "Whatever happens, happens." She leaves pregnancy up to happenstance. She does not seek medical advice or try any remedies when she fails to get pregnant after "doing it all the time." Mary and her husband give it a chance by forgoing birth control for six months. She then closes the window when pregnancy does not happen, quickly deciding that she does not want children anyway. Two months later, by chance (that fickle phenomenon), they lose the condom during sex and her period is late. She worries that she is pregnant and then is relieved to find out she is not, because by now she is certain that she did not want to be a mother. Mary does not mention God or any other supernatural forces, but she still symbolically restricts her own power to decide whether or not to become a mother. Chance is yet another route to "indecisions" about motherhood.

Pregnancy is unpredictable. Women try magical thinking, potions, charms, and rituals to prevent pregnancy and to achieve it. On one level they believe that God/the universe/ chance controls the situation, influences readiness and timing, and delivers karmic justice. But they do not rely on magic alone. The women I interviewed control their fertility in the sense that they have abortions, they use birth control, and they dabble to varying degrees in medical treatments to promote pregnancy. Because getting pregnant is an especially uncontrollable event in the lives of involuntarily childless women, constructing motherhood as an ascribed status, as God's blessing (or command), or as chance provides a comforting view. Women do not "decide" to be mothers: nature (or an omniscient, omnipotent power) does, and that is explanation enough.

For the women in this study, a perfect storm of readiness and divine influence gathers on its own to a large extent, and motherhood or childlessness is magically meant to be or supernatural but subject to influence (through positive thinking, trust in the universe, or "good vibes"). Yet God or fate or chance—not women and certainly not doctors—ultimately decides who will or will not become a mother and by which route.

6

REALIZATIONS

If we are to recognize and respect choice, we have to respect these choices as well: the choice to accept infertility and the choice to fight it.
—Barbara Katz Rothman, *Recreating Motherhood*

LaWanda Jackson, a forty-two-year-old nurse's aide, tells me that five years ago she did not want children but that she did not feel definite about that decision. More recently she began wanting children, but she volunteers—rather adamantly, in fact—that she never feels "desperate" about this new desire. Several of the women I spoke with make the outright claim that they are not desperate, that default image of infertile women.

Infertile, childless, or both, the women I interviewed relate their stories in ways that are ambiguous and inconsistent. Even if many of them express sadness, disappointment, or wistfulness at times, they generally describe these feelings as short-lived or diffuse. Some say they always wanted children but then go on to say that they maybe never really wanted them anyway. Some call themselves infertile but point out that there is still a chance they could get pregnant and have a baby. Some do not dwell on their childlessness; instead they declare themselves fulfilled, even as they weep during the interview for the lost opportunity to have grandchildren someday. Their feelings are complex.

Their so-called decisions are not firm ones. Their plans and their memories change even as they relate them to me.

Transcending Realizations

Recognizing one's infertility or involuntary childlessness is often not a discrete event. The study participants come to an awareness about their childlessness often unselfconsciously and gradually. Perceptions of fertility vary within one's lifetime, even within the conventionally defined fertile years (ages fifteen to forty-four). The women I spoke with discover in different ways that motherhood will not just happen for them and their reactions vary accordingly. For example, those for whom childlessness "just happened" cannot pinpoint when they realized that they were always going to be nonmothers.

Two outliers among the study participants, Azra Alic from Bosnia and Zara Senai from Eritrea, represent the most "infertile identified" of the women. They actively work to transcend the label of infertility. Azra, the only one pursuing ART (in the form of IVF), points out that when she was told that fertility could be a problem for her, "I wasn't thinking about kids at that time." She does not worry about her fertility potential when she first realizes that there could be a problem at the age of twenty-five. She is not yet interested in becoming a mother. She focuses on the abdominal pain she has and the need for surgical intervention. Her concern soon grows, however; and by the time I talk with her about it four years later, she is beginning IVF, feeling depressed and emotionally raw, and sullenly planning her future as a childless old maid. Only Azra and Zara, among my respondents, convey unresolved emotional pain in their interviews. These two women have much in common. Both endured large ovarian cysts and multiple surgeries, and both harbor doubt that their partners will still want them, despite reassurances of love and loyalty. Both women are secular Muslims who are fairly acculturated despite being first-generation immigrants. Zara keeps her uterus because, as she says, quoting her husband, "Maybe someday these people—they do a lot of research—something will come up; don't give up." These two women cherish their godmother auntie roles but see that as a second-best alternative to real motherhood. It took Azra a while to first realize that her fertility was in danger and that it was something she cared about. Now she is accepting medical treatment beyond her comfort level, leading me to wonder whether she is in fact getting a little bit desperate. However, she adamantly denies being "stressed" and indeed gets annoyed when doctors insinuate that she is. Both Azra and Zara clearly state that they know that there is more to life than motherhood and that they will eventually come to grips with that fact. They just have not done so yet.

Ambivalent Realizations

Several of the women vacillate between wanting children and not wanting children, sometimes in reaction to medical assertions regarding their fertility. They demonstrate their ambivalence by weighing the benefits and drawbacks of having children or not having them, by "wanting and not wanting" children at different points in their lives and at various times throughout the interview. This pattern holds true for the younger women who intentionally delay childbearing as well as for the women who have given up on the idea of having children or having additional children. By not making a clear distinction, the women allow for supernatural intervention, but they also leave open the possibility that they can and will change their minds and that there are other satisfactory paths in life besides being a mother:

> I think at one point [I wanted children] and then I
> found out I couldn't, so I was in denial about it, so it was
> more like, "Oh I don't want them anyway." And then I

really opened up [and began to want to have children] in my twenties. —*Jessie Silva, forty-two, white, queer, hair stylist*

I thought maybe I could never get pregnant. I think that the first two sexual experiences I ever had, I was not on the pill. And then I got on the pill. And I thought, "Gee, maybe I could never have children anyway." The story that comes to mind is my periods are getting further and further away. I thought I was pregnant from a boyfriend at age forty and I went to my doctor. I think I was starting to have hot flashes, too. And I went to my gynecologist and I said, "You know, I think I need something because—" I thought I was pregnant and he said, "No that's just your start of your peri-menopausal or whatever." And I go to say, "You mean I can't have children?" [*Disbelieving*] And it was weird because I think I had already said [to myself], "It's okay if you don't have children." But as soon as he said I can't, it was like, "What do you mean I *can't*?" And then he said, "Well, did you want to?" And I go, "Well, no, not really, because I'm not with anyone in my life that I could have the child with." —*Penny Ortiz, fifty-two, Latina, single, guidance counselor*

The threats to their self-concepts as women, to their assumption of fertility, to the options they thought they had about motherhood are serious but not determinative. As with any life-changing information, there are long-term pros and cons to consider and several possible directions to go. Jessie and Penny do not collapse upon hearing of their infertility, but neither do they take it in stride.

For other women, the realization sneaks up on them:

We finally got a house and then I had a new job and then it was like I had way too much responsibility. I guess I started trying then but I wasn't that serious. So probably around when I was thirty-eight I got more serious about trying. Suddenly I realized, maybe I'm not fertile anymore. —*Jennifer West, forty-six, Latina, married, engineer*

Many women recount the disorientation they felt when trying to get pregnant after many years of trying to prevent it. The fear of infertility supplants the fear of pregnancy. Jennifer remarks on the irony of this phenomenon. She "didn't really think about anything else" other than avoiding pregnancy, never considering that she might not ever have children someday. For her the realization came too late. She partly blames the media for her predicament, maintaining that her generation was brainwashed into delaying childbearing by amazing success stories and by older celebrity mothers on magazine covers. Once faced with the option of trying for a miracle, she realizes that she is unwilling to go through the medical ordeal. Jennifer ends up adopting an infant, a decision that she and her spouse come to incrementally—much more slowly, by comparison, than the other members of their cohort in the mandatory adoption-training classes they took.

Some women come to the realization that they will never be mothers when they awaken to the fact that they will never meet their own criteria of readiness. In fifty-six-year-old Lourdes Garcia's case, this realization happens somewhat suddenly. At the age of forty, she has her first and only sexual encounter, and it is a disappointment. As a result, she comes to understand that if she does not want an intimate relationship, then she will not have children. She talks a good deal about a close friend who adopted on her own, but Lourdes cannot reconcile herself to the lack of a partner with whom to raise children. Still, she entertains the idea throughout the interview, always coming to the conclusion that single motherhood is wrong for her.

Reflexive Realizations

Many of the women interviewed ponder the decisions they make—or decline to make—over their lifetimes and allow for ambiguity and the unpredictable unfolding of life events. They do not see infertility or childlessness as fixed statuses.

Sometimes women experience instances that disentangle fertility from motherhood:

> I realized that on a note card I had written "mother."
> I had not written "pregnant" and that was a real turn-
> around for me to realize, wait: my goal is to be a
> mother. . . . Well, I thought "mother" meant going
> through all this stuff. —*Dianne Jacobsen, fifty-six, white,
> single, life coach*

Over the course of several months, Dianne ponders her apparent infertility. She gets medical treatment for fibroids. She tries to be nice to her soon-to-be ex-husband when she is close to ovulation so that he will cooperate in her attempts to become pregnant. She stands on her head after sex to encourage sperm to swim into the fallopian tubes. She eventually finds out that her fallopian tubes are closed, signaling the end of her fertility. She writes herself reminder notes about her "goal." (Dianne fervently believes in self-help methods; she makes her living delivering motivational speeches and hiring herself out as a "life coach.") And then she realizes that "mother means you want to be a mother, not that you want to get pregnant." She wastes no time, signing up for adoption classes and a home study, exercises she enjoys for the self-examination they require. Finally, Dianne gets a call via her social connections about an available baby born thousands of miles away. She immediately flies out, takes the baby home, and soon thereafter divorces her husband, remaining single throughout the baby's childhood. In the personal lore of the adoptive mothers I talked with, realization usually led to action.

In contrast, some of the other women develop a wait-and-see attitude, not "realizing," not naming their "infertility." This viewpoint comes not out of superstition or the blush of finality on the word but out of the conviction that "infertile" fails to describe them:

> I personally don't know the reason why I don't have any children. I did want a child. I at one point was really trying very hard to get pregnant with a man that I live with now, that I've been with since 1991. And we were not able to. And he ended up having to go through some prostate surgery, so that meant that he was going to be sterile. —*Iris Hernandez, fifty-four, Latina, office assistant*

Iris never receives a diagnosis about her fertility, and she does not go so far as saving sperm for later insemination, for reasons that are unclear but may be related to moral doubts. She does not "know the reason" for her inability to get pregnant before her partner's prostate surgery. Like most of the respondents describing why they did not avail themselves of the available treatments, Iris uses hedge words like "kind of" to elide any underlying reasons, reasons she does not care to delineate even in her own mind. Later, she says, they "thought about" adoption, but it just did not "materialize." There is no clear explanation for that either, even though she notes ample opportunity to obtain an infant when she worked as clerk in a public maternity ward where newborns were abandoned on several occasions.

The women talk about ARTs in the same way these things are talked about in society at large, but they do not buy into the promises enough to promote these solutions to childlessness. Medicine makes it seem that all types of infertility as treatable.

There are no hopeless cases. Some chance of success exists thanks to the alphabet soup of available technologies—including IUI, ICI, HSG, IVF, GIFT, ZIFT, ICSI, and TESE—and the women I interviewed are aware of this fact. And there are always surrogacy arrangements in which people can even make use of their own gametes, preserving a genetic connection. (Incidentally, I found surrogacy arrangements to be shockingly routinized by the fertility clinics I contacted. Despite the well-publicized potential for future legal complications, at least two clinics include surrogacy in their bulleted list of services, and both mentioned it in phone consultations.)

It can seem unnecessary to think of oneself as "infertile" when it is always hypothetically possible to remedy the situation if the desire is great enough. Women can never really know how fertile they were in the past when using birth control or avoiding pregnancy in other ways, and they can never really know how fertile they are or will be in the future since they can never exhaust all possible remedies. Therefore, some women who are identified as infertile are infertile with caveats. Fertility fluctuates. These women apply the brakes themselves for personal and emotional reasons as well as for financial reasons:

> I should say it's not absolutely certain that I'm infertile.
> So part of the problem with this vague POF [premature
> ovulation failure] diagnosis is we don't know what it
> means. My ovaries aren't functioning properly, but
> since we don't know why, we don't know if they might
> start functioning again or what for the rest of my life,
> for the rest of my body. I think about 5 percent, or 5
> to 10 percent—I've seen different statistics—with POF
> eventually become pregnant. Sometimes twenty years
> after the diagnosis. So in saying I'm infertile, I'm just
> going with the statistical probability. And that's again not

something my doctor told me, but something I had to find out on my own. —*Hannah Johanson, thirty-nine, white, queer, married, teacher*

In Hannah's case, discouraged by the doctors' apparent lack of knowledge regarding her diagnosis, she casts a more critical eye on the medical establishment. She reexamines her (largely unconscious) acceptance of biologism and acknowledges that she *could* have biological, genetic children but that, given the circumstances, she prefers not to. She takes the power into her own hands by making adoption a deliberate choice, not merely the default option. And she can accept the label of infertility—in other words, become resigned to it—only once she sees other options for achieving motherhood. This is an important distinction because being called "infertile" is not acceptable until the resolution is in place either to mitigate the stigma or perhaps just to take the emotional sting out of a label that sounds so final. A woman can cop to being infertile if she is a mother anyway.

This pattern holds true not just for adoptive mothers but also for the women in the study experiencing secondary infertility. Forty-one-year-old Lupe Jimenez, who suffers repeated miscarriages, chooses to refocus her attentions on her existing child and to let go of the idea of producing a sibling for him. Her doctors suggest a new way to prevent her miscarriages, but she has had enough of the emotional turmoil and medical hoop jumping. She wants to "be happy" again and wants to sustain a healthy relationship with her son (who at the age of six, noting her sadness, reportedly reassures her, "It's okay if I don't have a brother or sister."). Doctors tell her she has a "weak" cervix, implying perhaps that she is somehow to blame for this lack of strength (see Martin 1987). But in spite of pressure from her doctors, her husband, and her mother (who constantly presses her to "try again"), Lupe refuses.

A clear transition from fertile to infertile (or to involuntary childlessness) does not necessarily happen among the women of this study who tend to be dubious about—if not outright opposed to—medicalization. For this reason, their experiences are too complex to map out the "reality reconstructions," "identity transformations," and "role readjustments" (Matthews and Matthews 1986) and the "redesigning the life plan" (Becker 2000) that some infertile women and couples go through (particularly after repeated failed IVF attempts). The "transition to nonparenthood" is less tangible because their goals are fuzzier in the first place and because they do not undergo the transformative immersion that happens with beginning, enduring, and then finally ending a rigorous treatment regimen. The women I talked with experience realizations about their infertility that remain in a state of flux. Even women like Iris and Mary, who have passed the menopausal stage, say they are unsure about whether they were infertile or whether or not they chose childlessness.

There are aspects of human biological reproduction that are unknown and, some suggest, unknowable, even by medical science. This missing knowledge helps fertility retain its mystery, leaving the door open for supernatural influences. It also leaves room for interpretation. Most women of childbearing age (an age that is creeping upward) see themselves as fertile or, at the very least, possibly fertile. The realization that one is infertile occurs along a continuum. It is a process. And this process can occur multiple times, in different ways each time, contingent on women's fluctuating biology, changing social circumstances, and temporally situated psychological and emotional states.

Coping and Regret

Thankfully, I now have two healthy and happy sons whom we were able to adopt. I go about my everyday business of writing this book, caring for the children, managing a household, teaching, and keeping up with other social, professional, and familial obligations, barely remembering my own "devastation" from infertility. (I no doubt belonged on that end of the spectrum with women who approximate the stereotype of the desperate infertile determined to achieve motherhood.) But I felt differently in the summer of 2006 when I finally—after six years of trying—realized that my fertility pursuit was over and that we would try to adopt. Here is an excerpt from a journal entry jotted down immediately after talking with the clinic nurse over the phone:

> Today 7/21/06 I had the nurse consultation with the Zouves clinic. She detailed the procedures for precycle testing in which I would have to be tested for hormone levels, immune responses, psychological counseling (because we are using donor sperm), and genetic counseling and tests (even though we are using pre-screened donor sperm). The medications will total into the thousands, the counseling fees are not listed on their lists of fees (which already total about 30K), and there are required shots daily for about four months. Some shots are twice daily, etc. I feel that I can't do it because if it doesn't work it will be torture for nothing (but more torture in an emotional sense), will require lots of time off work in my untenured position, and will max out our credit. . . .

> Now I feel upset, maybe even devastated (at least within the hour of the phone call) that I will not experience a pregnancy and birth. I cried. . . . IVF is not indicated, only in the sense that IUI hasn't worked for so long. That miscarriage was not about the method (ICI/IUI

versus IVF) but about proper medical monitoring. Perhaps I just need a good doctor. . . . One thing that makes me feel better even though I am sad about the idea that I may well not get to experience a pregnancy is that I may still get to breastfeed. I need to look into how that is done for foster/adoptive moms. . . . The physical experience is a small and perhaps forgettable part of that in the scheme of my lifetime or my child's lifetime. I am beginning to feel less scared of adoption and less loss about IVF and the imagined pregnancy (not even the baby, in fact. It's the pregnancy I am mourning).

In this passage, I work through my thoughts in an attempt to cope with the loss, coming to the conclusion that adoption will heal me, or correct the "disability" of infertility (Rothman 2000b, 95), especially if I still get to embody motherhood through breastfeeding (I *was* able to breastfeed the second child). The coping stories among my respondents echo my own in some key ways: expressions of sadness or regret, questions of blame, frustration at loss of power via doctors' presumed ineptitude, critiques of medicalization and "society," glorification of the pregnancy experience, and, of course, resolution through some other plan (or, for some, through giving up planning altogether). It may be overreaching to use the term "cope." For so many, it is a gradual, irresolute process, a phenomenon that goes hand in hand with indefinite, ephemeral realizations. Hedge words and phrases—like "maybe," "I guess," "probably," and "sort of"—litter the speech of even the most contented of the respondents in describing their comfort with their infertility or childlessness. This practice indicates a little uncertainty and shows that coping must be continually negotiated. My conversations with these women yield some patterns that vary in intensity. Generally speaking, the childless women find good reasons to be that way even while they express mild to moderate longing or regret. I talked to them at disparate points in the coping process in part because of where they happen to be along the life course.

Not Meeting Expectations

Even the women who lean toward identifying as voluntarily childless must contend with their choice within an entrenched pronatalist society:

> I'm not sure [if I wanted children]. I thought I did. But in retrospect, I think it was more just doing what my older sisters did and what my mother did. . . . I remember thinking that I would at least go to college and get a degree and then I'd have kids. . . . I decided somewhere along the line to not [have children]. I don't think it was ever really conscious. It was conscious when I thought I was going to have kids at nineteen or twenty because I was with a guy that wanted kids and we were talking about all these kids. But then that fell apart and then I never really thought about it. . . . We'd have a bunch of kids because he liked kids and I liked kids. So it was pretty flip. It wasn't in any depth at all. . . . The only thing I think about is who's going to take care of me when I'm eighty-five. Now that I work with seniors, I wish I'd had kids! I don't really think about it. I kid around with you that I wish I had kids. —*Annette Kramer, fifty-four, white, lesbian, family therapist*

Annette's comments mirror those of the other postmenopausal childless women; she cannot pinpoint a time when she decided not to have children, nor was her earlier plan to have them ever serious in this telling. This indecisiveness about motherhood and her levity suggest minimum regret. Other older women I spoke with by and large appear content with their lives and their choices; they often say that they "don't dwell" on their childlessness. This is not to suggest that they lack awareness of their erstwhile deviance. Annette, for example, recounts a recent uncomfortable incident wherein others were apparently "judging" her because she did not have children (she was certain they would have been positively shocked to learn that she was also a lesbian). Karen related a similar event: "When I think about it, I think it's strange, and people must think I'm a little odd." She is a little surprised herself:

> By the time I was forty, I just said it looks like it's not going to happen. But it *is* weird to me. I've been thinking of it the last few years because it seems like I should have them in a way. I love my nieces and nephews and my friends' kids, but it feels strange like I could have also have had the life with the family. I don't sit around regretting it, but sometimes I think that's weird. It's weird that I didn't have [children]. —*Karen Tabb, forty-nine, white, single, teacher*

It is not until Karen is nearly fifty, long after she first accepts her childlessness, that she needs to actively cope. During our interview, Karen begins to cry when thinking about what could have been. This emotional response stuns her as she never had explored these latent feelings, earlier conveying some emotional distance by marveling at how "weird" it was that someone like herself, who loves children, never actually had any. She was among those who thanked me for the "free therapy," and she later e-mails me again to express gratitude for the catharsis.

The women in their childbearing years experience pressure to meet social expectations by becoming mothers, and they also predict how they will feel in the future if they remain nonmothers at other points along the standard life course. A couple of the middle-aged lesbians told me that they do not feel it is expected within their social circles to become mothers but that they often have to out themselves to explain their childlessness to strangers. Younger lesbians and queer women are arguably more beholden to the newer, more inclusive motherhood mandate that assumes all women, not just those partnered with men, will become mothers (Agigian 2004; Mamo 2007). Indeed, several of the single women, whose childlessness is largely attributable to being unattached, report that not having children causes the greater dissonance in social interactions. This pattern holds true even among the Latinas I interviewed, for whom marriage and children, they say, must come in that order. They struggle to navigate emotionally the contradictory expectations that they should be mothers but that they should not be single mothers.

Altering the Life Course

The speed at which women arrive at resolution depends on many factors: their age and life-course stage, social status (e.g., married or single, poor or middle class), drive to become mothers, degree of medicalization, and idiosyncratic events. Sadness or regret may last a month or a year, or may crop up here and there throughout their lifetime. Mary, for example, never minded her childlessness one whit, firmly concluding within a six-month period in her twenties that pregnancy was just not going to happen and that she did not want children anyway. Much later, a spate of events shifts her perspective:

> We go, "Oh, okay, let's have kids," and we tried but we didn't have any. And then, "I don't want any kids right now." We were free. We could do what we wanted. So then we were fine. And then about a year ago, I started

freaking out. Like, "Oh why didn't I have kids?" Oh yeah.
I was going through it for a couple of months. Every time
somebody would ask, "What was the one thing you most
regretted in life?" And I'd go, "Not having kids." And I'd
burst into tears. But now I'm like okay again [laughs].

Kristin Wilson: What brought that on, do you think?

All my friends were having grandkids now. And I'm the
only one that doesn't have any kids at all. They'd go,
"Oh, do you want to go to a baby shower?" I went to many
baby showers and then I started thinking one day and I
got in that rut and I cried about it every time someone
asked me. . . . And then I was thinking, I don't have
any kids. I won't have any grandkids. But now I see my
friends and they have teen kids and they struggling now
because, "Oh, I've got to send him to college and I can't
afford to do this." And then I'm thinking, "I'm lucky
because I don't have to provide for that." —*Mary Benson,
forty-eight, African American, married, cook*

Mary goes almost a quarter of a century without worrying about
her childlessness, and then it hits her. The mourning is acute
but brief. Now she laughs about what she characterizes as her
earlier histrionics. Her experience illustrates that the meaning
of childlessness changes throughout the life course and that
women constantly renegotiate their feelings and identities with
each new encounter. Put together, these insights challenge truisms about childlessness and infertility. Childless women are
not insouciantly childfree, nor are they lonely old maids.

Intersecting Strategies
Most of the women employ multiple strategies for explaining
themselves:

I thought I was never going to get pregnant. Sometimes I was okay about it. Oh, good, my husband doesn't want to have children. But, sometimes I was kind of sad. Because my husband was in his own world and I was basically alone. I could do whatever I want, but then you know there was some point that you said, "Oh, look at those children in the park and they're playing; oh, I wish I could have one." —*Serena Lopez, thirty-nine, Latina, married, pharmacy technician*

I met Serena and her two-year-old, slightly developmentally delayed son in an empty courtyard at a library near San Jose, California. Her fertility history reveals how women can both accept and regret their infertility many times. She says that "sometimes [she] was okay about it" when she could not get pregnant with her first husband. She enjoys traveling and the freedom to do what she wants. Toward the end of their marriage—in a decision that is indeed the cause of its demise—he declares that he cannot in good conscience add another child to a society run aground. His work with "juvenile delinquents" leads to this conclusion, instigating Serena's request for a divorce, because at an undefined point, she begins yearning for children like those she observes at the park. While single, she becomes very close to a friend for whom she acts as childbirth coach and, later, frequent babysitter. This role sustains her for a good while.

After some time, she takes up with a man who is already a father, and they talk about having children together someday. Although she feels pressure from her boss, her friends and acquaintances, and her mother to "hurry up" before she ages out of her fertility, she resists this pressure, saying that she is not ready, as she wants to finish school and buy a house. Finally, she tries to get pregnant but to no avail for over a year, and so then seeks medical help. She takes Clomid and does get pregnant, but ends up with preeclampsia, other complications, and a premature baby born weighing barely over one pound. She is saddened by her secondary infertility—really a decision not to risk complications again—but also implies that one child is quite enough for her. However, she and her new husband discuss adoption frequently, though she fears giving preferential treatment to her biological child.

Serena readily adapts her thinking as her situation changes. She tries every tack by turns: appreciating a childfree lifestyle while honoring her then-husband's preference, pursuing other life goals, becoming a godmother auntie, using assisted conception, considering adoption, and asserting that she could not handle two children anyway (particularly in light of her son's special needs). Coping and regret are ever present, but they are nebulous feelings. Women go back and forth between the two phenomena, depending on what is going on in their lives.

Take into account the following comments from two women using ARTs, one of whom is critical of medicalization:

> If I'm not to have kids, what can I do? I'm not the only one you know. It's hard but . . . I think I'm ready to have kids. And I was ready a long time. And my partner is ready and that's what everybody's suggesting. Everywhere I went, I had a few opinions on everything. Everything seems okay, everything seems to be working, but there is something wrong inside since I'm not getting pregnant. And they're saying, "You do the IVF process, you will skip it." . . . I mean if I have to adopt my kids, I'd love them the same but still I would like to have my own kids. I don't know how to explain that. —*Azra Alic, thirty, engaged, apartment manager*

> We're open to adoption but we can't really get too open to it. My partner and I talk about it not a lot, but

enough. She says, "I'd be really open to adoption." And I feel as the one trying to get pregnant, a little more reserved about opening up to it too much. I feel like if I were open to it, I'd be telling my body something. "No, I want [my body] to work for it!" There's something psychological. Maybe if I was more open, my body would feel less pressure. I feel like I don't know what that's about. It's all these questions. This maddening thing. — *Robin Smith, forty-two, white, lesbian, fertility counselor*

Adoption is on the table for Azra, though she prefers to have her own children, while Robin cannot let herself ponder that option when she is still trying to get pregnant, lest she tempt fate. Infertility and childlessness are always in the process of being reconciled. Azra and Robin, while intensifying their attempts to get pregnant, try on assorted narratives. For instance, Azra thinks perhaps she could leave it up to fate like so many other women must do, and she contends that adoption could work for her and—elsewhere in the interview—she notes satisfaction in being a godmother auntie, and all the while she maintains her commitment to getting pregnant even if she has to resort to IVF, a process she abhors. She may be able to get pregnant without Clomid and IVF, but she submits to treatment not because her doctors suggest it but because she feels time is running out for her. By bringing up adoption and other possibilities, Azra prepares for what some infertility researchers call "reality reconstruction," a reimagining of what they want in life (Matthews and Matthews 1986).

Coping for the women who are not yet ready to have children is about coming up with a future plan that balances all their other needs with the desire to be mothers. Some are in the midst of accepting that there may be a problem. Others have comfortably reconciled their situation. Close examination of the words of this latter group reveals lingering ambivalence, however. For example, Penny says, "Maybe it was a blessing that I didn't have children because what did he get to do for his daughter?" She alludes to her ex-husband's discovery of a daughter late in his life. Following his divorce with Penny, he became involved with her friend, who got pregnant and then put their daughter up for adoption. When the girl reached adulthood, she located the father, and he ended up giving her away at her wedding, thus beginning a lasting, warm relationship. Penny rapturously tells this touching story that illustrates how her childlessness was meant to be in the universal scheme of things.

There are ways to get past even very negative feelings about infertility and childlessness:

> Probably my ovaries only stopped working in my thirties, a few months before I was diagnosed. It's really hard to know. Maybe around thirty, maybe thirty-two, maybe closer to thirty-four when I was diagnosed. And again, this didn't last very long, but at first I was very, very mad at myself for having waited because I may well have been fertile prior to my thirties. And I talked with Adriana [my female partner, with whom I seriously considered having children when we were both in our twenties] about a lot of these things, that if I had children instead of waiting and making other life decisions, that if I'd tried having biological children earlier, the infertility part wouldn't matter. Again, pretty quickly that was a nonissue. —
> *Hannah Johanson, thirty-nine, white, queer, married, teacher*

Hannah recalls her swiftly dismissed but strongly felt self-blame at the decision to put off childbearing. She ultimately settles these regrets in two complementary ways: emotionally and intellectually through feminist introspection, and practically by successfully adopting a child and achieving her preeminent goal of motherhood. She connects her experience to wider societal patterns such as those that force the nonchoice between higher education and career pursuits and motherhood during the most fertile years. Hannah, who happened to be in training to become a therapist during this time, also analyzes her feelings and methodically separates her health concerns from her assumptions about femininity, and motherhood from her mind-set about aging prematurely (because of early menopause). Adopting a daughter from China, a course that unleashed a roller-coaster ride of emotion, eventually transformed Hannah's daily experience from hopeful and anxious to busy and fulfilled.

Not everyone has the luxury of Hannah's well-honed emotional tools. But the women I interviewed, who come from many walks of life, tend to find equilibrium between their acceptance and their regret regardless of where I found them in their "journey." This capability comes from their ability to realize their situations from different angles over time and to draw on flexible coping strategies. They decline the label "infertile" and all that would connote about their experiences and their lives. They make their own meanings.

INTERVENTIONS

The women of this study rarely mention the moral concerns that are sometimes part of the public debate about ARTs. Other people worry about the personhood of embryos, the unknown health consequences for women, and the dangers of creating Franken-babies. Feminists voice fears about unfettered pronatalism and about the negative impacts and false promises of medicalization. And it is access to treatment that is often the primary worry for public health advocates who decry the prohibitive cost and clinics' subtle and overt discrimination against marginalized groups who might otherwise benefit from ARTs.

The women tell me instead that they do not seek treatment because they—as individuals, not as members of a particular group—do not "fit in." A discourse of difference shapes these women's personal stories and allows them to disregard some social norms that dictate how women should be. They end up largely rejecting those interventions—medical treatment and adoption—that promise to make (other) childless or infertile women normal.

Not Fitting In

At times, the study participants embrace the deviance of childlessness as evidence of their singular qualities. Many claim to be individually "different" in that they "don't follow the crowd," they are "shy" or "reserved," and they display fierce "independence," as if these characteristics explain their childlessness or infertility:

> All of my older sisters are married. But being the little one, I am the travel person in the family, the one who has more curiosity about life and adventure. And just being different in that way, and I was the first one to have a job outside my father's business. I [am] more independent and aggressive in life. —*Lourdes Garcia, fifty-six, Latina, single, office assistant*

Being Too Independent

Separate from the idea of not fitting in, but very closely related to it, is the notion of "being too independent." It is a stance or a declaration about these women's abilities to make life choices for themselves as well as a personality trait that makes one less feminine and, consequently, less suitable for motherhood. This attitude can be a point of pride in a society that values independence writ large:

> I think it [not wanting children] goes back to being independent early on. Being one of eleven, you really had to take care of yourself. So there was that early independence that led me to hold my own ideas independently. Sometimes too independently, actually! —*Annette Kramer, fifty-four, white, lesbian, family therapist*

Annette and another woman I interviewed, Lana Marks, a fifty-two-year-old lesbian and nurse, both note that they associate mainly with other childless lesbian couples. They marvel a bit about all the lesbians now starting families, something they describe as an acceptable—but confounding—life choice. One could argue that they embrace a masculinist model of women's liberation in that their focus is on their careers and they have female partners who take on more of the domestic duties. They are less involved nonmothers and see motherhood as too limiting, too conventional. To them, caring for children is a role other kinds of (slightly duped) women take on. Lana wonders why they do not just get a dog to satisfy their needs to nurture.

They characterize themselves as antithetical to men's expectations, as reflective of a femininity that does not require them to be mothers. This is not the case for all of the lesbians and sexual minorities I interviewed. Lourdes, for instance, who brings up her sexuality at the end of the interview when I fail to ask about it, tells me that some people question her sexuality, tying her childlessness to suspected lesbianism. She specifically blames her childlessness on her independent spirit, describing herself as perhaps overly masculine. Lourdes sometimes rejects the idea that "to be a woman is to be a mother," but she seems to hang on to some inward critiques about her own femininity as a childless, single woman, not interested in men and thus prohibited from motherhood.

Feeling Less a Woman

Other women feel left out and less feminine specifically due to their infertility:

> I don't think you ever get over the sadness because there's so much that comes with not—I think it's all head stuff. Not feeling like a woman. I think I was just feeling so imbalanced all the time and I mean like my periods not starting and now I haven't had a period since I was thirty years old . . . I stopped. My story just didn't connect with all of the people I met. So feeling just really alone.
> —*Jessie Silva, forty-two, white, queer, hair stylist*

Unlike Lourdes, Jessie does not conflate femininity with sexuality. She finally, somewhat magically in her telling, becomes a mother via adoption, thus fulfilling her feminine destiny and resolving her loneliness. In Jessie's case, the fact that her story "just didn't connect" with others encourages her to act in nonconformist ways such as adopting a child without a partner.

Jessie's self-esteem problems compel her to work on herself. This kind of introspection, influenced by not fitting in, comes up in many of the interviews. Several of the African American women bring up colorism. Being either too dark-skinned or too light-skinned leads to merciless teasing, loneliness, lack of confidence, and mistrust of men. These experiences partially account, they say, for their childlessness.

LaWanda's story is particularly traumatic. Her mother sent her to live in a foster home and kept her other four children. LaWanda thinks that her mother disliked her because of her light skin since it favored that of her father, her mother's estranged partner. She spent years searching for self-esteem through multiple failed marriages. Now she wants a child in part because she finally feels more self-assured (also because she thinks it is her Christian duty and because she wants to be admired). Two of the young women I talked with, Nicole and Shana, delayed childbearing to "get themselves right" by amassing self-respect and maturity through work and education in order to heal their emotional wounds. They talk about how they will mother a child (always assumed to be a daughter) with skin like or different from theirs, insisting that they will love them and inculcate them with the self-esteem needed to confront daily slights and judgments rooted in colorism. They are wary of the attentions of men right now, and although they expect to get married and have children "someday," they think informal—and perhaps formal—adoption might work for them should they not find the right relationship. Being marked as different by their peers impacts their self-defined readiness for motherhood.

Some of the women feel inadequately feminine. Part of this thinking involves the belief that only fully fledged women can be real moms but, in a bit of a catch-22, one must already be a mother to be a complete woman. To attempt to reach this balance, several women are working toward improving their self-regard in order to ensure readiness for motherhood and also to attract supernatural intervention that might lead to motherhood. The women who have given up on motherhood, of course, do not talk like this. Instead, they proclaim, sometimes defensively, that they are real women despite their childlessness.

Defending Difference

The childless women I talked with encounter misdirected pity and inevitable suspicion by those they encounter in the course of everyday life. Some of the women can satisfactorily explain their childlessness by outing themselves as lesbians, though they tire of the nosy questions. Those who adopted children also have to defend their choice, usually by constructing it as preferable and preordained, even if they went the adoption route only after first attempting to enter motherhood more conventionally via pregnancy and childbirth.

Several of the young African American women I interviewed endorse a mainstream (white) point of view, a position they have to defend:

> The school I came from, most of the girls there have
> kids or are pregnant now. [My best friend] and I was just
> talking about that the night before last. Saying how when
> we see people we used to go to high school with, they'll be
> like, "Where your baby at?" And it's like, "I don't have any
> children." "Oh, you ain't got no baby daddy?" "No." "You

ain't got no boyfriend?" "That's none of your business if I do. I'm just telling you I don't have children, I don't have no kids, I'm not responsible for no one but myself." — *Jamilah Washington, nineteen, African American, single, student*

They have an attitude. They look down on me because they feel I feel that I'm better than them. And I don't. I just didn't have a baby. I don't look down on you because you had a baby. It was the decision you made. It was something you did. And I don't think you should look down on me because I'm succeeding and prospering in life and doing well, and that's not to say you can't either.
—*Nicole Lambert, twenty, African American, single, student*

These women are young and unattached, and these interviews reflect their thinking at a point in time. Should love or other life events intervene, they may change their minds quickly as they have a counterdiscourse available to them that equates adulthood with motherhood and presumes that twenty-five is old for becoming a mother. From this insider/outsider position, they have a kind of freedom in that they can easily tap into a supporting narrative, whichever outcome occurs.

Unique Points of View
Several of the study participants refer to having special insights that allow them greater reflexivity and a capacity to cope more effortlessly with the disruption of infertility or childlessness. Some attribute their resilience and perspective to loneliness, being a "spiritual seeker," or having been treated for depression and other neuroses:

I have social anxiety disorder or whatever you call it. I start to freak out, have panic attacks in big crowds. So I have to limit myself to just being with two or three people. I like to be in control, but that's not the most important thing. I would rather have a peaceful group than a group that has a lot of dissent but I'm in control. —*Annie Adoyo, thirty, second-generation African immigrant, single, student*

Annie wants to make her way in the world on her own terms. She admits to having some previous problems with handling her finances and with functioning on a day-to-day basis. But through counseling and mood-enhancing pharmaceuticals, she has arrived at a good place within herself. Motherhood is a duty or vocation she feels called to perform despite the fact that she is single and underemployed. She is unconcerned about finding the right partner or the right time—an unusual attitude among my respondents.

Talia, who is Jewish by birth, dabbles in Christianity (a larger than life-sized portrait of Jesus hangs above her bed in her studio apartment, where we had our interview), Buddhism, and New Age mysticism, all traditions she draws on extensively in trying to get her body "ready" for pregnancy even though she does not have a partner. She muses about calling a sperm bank soon since she is approaching her mid-forties. Emily, on the other hand, thinks having a child will give her something constructive to do and prevent her from wallowing in loneliness or watching too much television, previous habits that instigated a prescription for antidepressants and getting involved in foster care.

The women's supposed intrinsic differences provide them with somewhat off-kilter points of view by which to examine and renegotiate the inherent promises of social ideas about motherhood, infertility, childlessness, and treatment. They do not fit societal expectations, and so maybe the expected ways of doing things will not work for them. They are in some ways freer to forge different paths in life, to deftly cope with and defend their decisions.

Medical Interventions

The foremost purpose of medically assisted conception (and, arguably, adoption) is to redress the handicap of childlessness. Yet, for a variety of reasons, most of the women who participated in this project have not become lured by this siren call. They hear it, to be sure; indeed, the existence of ARTs impacts them considerably. For example, it allows them to "settle down" before even thinking of having children, as one woman put it.

Yet, from their standpoints at the social margins, the women I talked with are more apt to doubt the assumptions of the medical (and adoption) worlds. They exercise this "epistemic privilege" (Collins 1991, 1999) by dismissing what doctors tell them and sometimes by using medicine and adoption selectively to their own advantage, ignoring attempts to get them on the "infertility treadmill" (Harwood 2007).

QUESTIONING THE EXPERTS

Some do not like doctors and medicine because they neither understand nor trust them:

> He basically said—and this was a urologist—he suggested doing something about saving the sperm, freezing the sperm, but I don't think anything was very clear. . . . How would the results affect the child? It wasn't very clear and I think that maybe I didn't really, maybe we didn't really, when we saw that there were some obstacles, we just didn't pursue it. —*Iris Hernandez, fifty-four, Latina, office assistant*

This couple's confusion led to the decision not to preserve their potential for fertility.

Whereas I suspect that overriding Iris's interest in having a baby were concerns over her partner's prostate cancer, the reported interaction with the doctor reveals an ideological chasm between the promises of assisted conception and a woman's belief in those promises. Saving sperm, to the doctor, is a simple procedure as is the subsequent insemination. It happens every day and requires no medication, no surgery, and, truth be told, no special medical knowledge (I did this at home myself). Refracted through the lens available to Iris, however, it becomes one with those mysterious, cutting-edge, almost sci-fi, technomedical experiments. She does not want to know, and so she does not pursue it.

Some of the women rail against the insensitivity of doctors. Medical personnel frustrate the women in their inability to understand that the knowledge they share, the test results they provide, have real-world ramifications with the potential to destroy life plans and challenge the core of their patients' identity:

> [The doctor] told me over the phone that I was in fact in menopause. She used the term menopause although medically that's not correct, and told me that that meant I was infertile, and then said goodbye! So I was basically told over the phone. She did nothing to prepare me; it was just a call on the phone. I was utterly devastated. . . . I think what was going through my head was that we couldn't have children. And we'd made a lot of decisions, we'd done a lot of planning, we'd talked a lot about how our lives would be with children. . . . I don't know why I couldn't begin to think about other options, but for a while I really couldn't. It just felt like we wouldn't have children. And part of that is actually part of the phrasing. . . . People will say, "You can't have children." And that's sort of something that people will talk about if they're talking about POF [premature ovulation

failure]. . . . What in fact is meant in my case is that I was infertile and could not bear a child in the traditional way biologically. —*Hannah Johanson, thirty-nine, white, queer, married, teacher*

Hannah, whose class status and educational attainment enhance her "cultural health capital" (Mamo 2007), seriously researches and considers the medical options but ultimately decides that those choices will not work in her particular case. She does not dismiss medical and scientific knowledge per se. In fact, she participates in experimental treatment on the other side of the country in hopes that clinicians will discover some sort of cure for POF.

Others, particularly the poor and working-class women and the women of color, question medical authority more fundamentally:

In terms of kids, I was pretty much thinking the same, that I don't want kids. Probably not until maybe about twenty-five, thirty at the most. Only because at a certain age you cannot bear kids. But my grandmother had my mother when she was forty-two. My grandmother had my mother during the change of life. . . . So I guess with medical [*sic*] saying "that-is-that" after a certain age, like thirty-five, it's going to be harder for you to bear kids. But, being that my grandmother had [my mother] in her early forties, sometime I kind of think it's possible, and one of my cousin's friends just also had a baby and she's forty-two. So like, I'm starting to wonder, are they really saying, is what medical [is] saying, is it really true? Or is it just because they were fortunate enough to have kids at that age? —*Shana Jones, twenty-five, African American, single, student*

Shana's skepticism highlights the gap between scientific knowledge and personal experience. Medical advice is convincing only if it squares with what she already knows or can see evidence for in her own life. Still, the fertility nosedive said to begin at age thirty-five jibes with her plan to have children by age thirty "at most." At twenty-five, she is already at the age that she thought she would be having children. But she is single and underemployed, still living with her mother, under her mother's rules. Because she cannot envision having a child in these circumstances, she wonders about the possibility of fertility in her early forties if it should come to that.

Several of the women I spoke with are dubious about doctors' motivations in offering assisted conception, especially ARTs:

> Yeah, [I would consider IVF] if I had the money and a partner. It's very expensive. And I don't know why they make it so difficult for women who want to have babies. I can see a couple thousand. But to throw ten, twenty thousand dollars to do that is just mad! Can't these doctors have compassion? . . . They want to be rich. How technical could the procedure be? It's not like open heart surgery or taking out a gall bladder. And then they're taking the sperm and whatever they do with the equipment. —*Talia Stein, forty-one, white, single, home healthcare aide*

> And then when I went to my new doctor, she asked me, "Have you ever been pregnant? Do you want to be pregnant?" and whatever. She went on this high-horse thing about, "If you ever want to get pregnant, just let me know." She says, "I have fabulous doctors I can send you." She goes, "Matter of fact, I'm pregnant now." I mean she went off. And I thought, how disrespectful. I just felt like

this is not what I'm here for. I'm here for my annual Pap, not to be sold a child. It was weird. That's how I saw her communicating with me. —*Penny Ortiz, fifty-two, Latina, single, guidance counselor*

Whether the women I interviewed see the doctors withholding treatment from those who want it or pushing it on those who do not, the doctors appear self-interested and lacking in compassion. Talia and Penny are angry that medicine is not what it purports to be. It is neither the manifestation of scientific progress nor a healing art.

The women in this study, for the most part, are not targeted and not fooled by industry advertising that portrays assisted conception as an improvement over nature. They buy into the convention that SNAF families produce children through heterosexual intercourse as an "expression of their love." Iris Hernandez encapsulates the sentiment that several of the women express: "When you have a marriage and you have a father and a mother for that child. I think that's beautiful."

Even as they see "having your own" as ideal, in choosing childlessness or adoption and skipping most medical options, the women I talked with challenge the idea that motherhood is for every woman.

THE ART (OF) HORROR STORIES
Cautionary tales about infertility and medicalization serve to explain why some respondents abstain from (further) assisted conception techniques:

> My sister went through all of that. And I said, I'm not going to do that. I saw what it did to her. Not only just emotionally, but she went through—I'm trying to think how many—artificial, in vitro, multiple times. It was just

like, I don't think I'll do that. Emotional. She would get hugely bloated ovaries when she was taking shots. The disappointment when it didn't work. She would be devastated. She's two years older than I am. I got married before she did. I think she would prefer that it didn't happen that way. And then I had a child before she did. . . . I feel that she didn't bond with [my son] because she was on these meds and she wasn't supposed to hold anything heavy, so she would not hold him! It'd be like, you have to be that careful with your body when you're going through treatments—that you can't hold a baby. Or it makes you upset to hold a baby. So I didn't want to go on that roller coaster. And financially, we're not in the same place my sister is. She's quite well off. So they can do that. It was probably seven in vitros that they did. Yeah. Yeah. And artificials and everything else. And I don't do well with the pelvic exams. They're usually very painful, they're uncomfortable. I don't want people doing that [to me]. —*Aikiko Moto, forty-three, Japanese American, married, teacher*

Another woman, Lupe Jimenez, has a traumatic miscarriage, which finally convinces her to stop trying for a second child. The experience becomes even more horrible when the nurses mistreat her because they mistakenly think she is suffering from a botched abortion. Though she credits her doctor with saving her from the nasty nurses, the general tone of her account is negative ("they pumped me full of medicine"). Both of these women can be described as having secondary infertility, although each stresses that she *could* birth another baby if she were committed to really "trying." But they want to avoid ill treatment as well as additional physical and emotional pain. A certain feeling of powerlessness permeates their stories. An individual doctor may be a heroic savior, but the overall experience is alienating and painful. They put a stop to treatment early on despite the many pressures to continue.

TAKING CONTROL

Instead of letting medicine be done *to* them, some women have medical treatment done *for* them, on their own terms:

> Well, realistically, I'm forty. And I went to this famous intuitive psychic. She's a medical intuitive, and from what people say, she's pretty accurate. I said, "What do you see for me down there?" She says, "Well, you're healthy down there. You can get pregnant. That's not the problem. The problem is that you have a higher chance of getting a Down's syndrome baby." And I was like, "Oh, gee." But from what this lady said, we're born with so many eggs, and what happens is you get three thousand or something like that. You still have a lot when you're older but some of them are dormant, and have to open up or something like that, she explained to me. —*Talia Stein, forty-one, white, single, home healthcare aide*

Talia puts more stock in the spiritual side of life than in science, despite the fact that she has medical training. She also lacks health insurance and so decides to take herbs to help "open up" her dormant eggs. However, she does not have a clear idea about where the sperm will come from. She considers a sperm bank, "hooking up" with someone from Craigslist, and getting pregnant by her new boyfriend without his knowledge. Failing these possibilities, she may adopt. Pairing medical-scientific knowledge about oocyte depletion with supernatural intervention (four respondents mentioned visiting psychics specifically to understand their infertility) is one way to undermine medical authority while taking advantage of its benefits. This route also helps individualize and make spiritual one's path to motherhood.

Sometimes women, especially those with relatively more social power, take control within highly medicalized contexts like surgery:

> They removed twenty-eight fibroids from my uterus, which was a record! And they were infertility specialists. So my whole uterus was kind of shredded after that. But *I really empowered them* [*emphasis added*] before the surgery. When they came in to talk with me before the surgery, I said, "Just remember that the reason we're going through this is that I want to get pregnant. It's not that the fibroids hurt. We wouldn't even be going through this surgery if I weren't trying to get pregnant. So if at all possible, if you could save my uterus, and everything else, that would be a really good thing." So they saved the uterus. —*Dianne Jacobsen, fifty-six, white, single, life coach*

To Dianne the authority is hers, not theirs, as it is her body being operated on for the fulfillment of her desire to become a mother.

A degree away from this empowered patient is the patient as full-fledged consumer. The women in this study, though neither fully immersed nor invested in the medicalized world of fertility treatment, still cast themselves hypothetically as prospective buyers. Much in the way that regular people idly dream of purchasing the million-dollar homes in those free real-estate magazines once found at newspaper stands, some women browse sperm donor catalogs:

> [The donor I chose] has blue eyes, which is a big thing. The other thing is, he has a negative blood type, and a

lot of the donors that they have there have positive blood types, and I'm O-neg, so I figure that helps make things easier, since you do get to pick. And he doesn't have any red flags. Some of the donors have red flags, as far as in their medical histories. He's a young college student, as a lot of them are. He wrote a little bit about why he's doing that, and I liked the reasons that he said. He's very kind-hearted. —*Emily Reilly, thirty, white, single, fast food restaurant manager*

I talk to my friends about it all the time. I say, we'll go up to San Francisco and look through the catalog. You see all these good qualities and everything that the men have—seven feet tall [*laughs*], or blue eyes, whatever it is. But everyone has an ugly relative. So just because you are reading all this doesn't guarantee you anything. And it's just pretty much like having your own kid. I mean, you've seen really good-looking parents out there with not so good-looking kids. And I hate to say that, but I've seen some ugly kids. —*Annie Adoyo, thirty, second-generation African immigrant, single, student*

Either one of these women might actually pursue donor insemination, but they are not yet committed to doing so. They shop with a discerning eye, one tinged with eugenic fantasies, yet in identifying the irony of a weird process that carries no guarantee, these women reveal their misgivings. Their taste in sperm donors reflects positively on them. The women in this study are perhaps not the ones to whom these catalogs specifically cater—sociologist Katherine Johnson (2009) shows how single women are subtly discouraged—but they are by no means immune to the allure. Practically speaking, they want to become mothers, and for women without partners, sperm banks provide a necessary product. In addition, their (imagined) use of sperm banks is decidedly liberating for the simple fact that these women are intending to have babies intentionally outside of the SNAF norm.

Although the turkey-baster method is technically simple, medical discourses make it sound perilous, especially because of fears of HIV transmission. And doctors tout better statistical chances with doctor-performed IUI (intrauterine insemination) than at-home ICI (intracervical insemination). These supposed benefits may be cast to coincide with a consumer's desire to have the best. And having the best is a big deal in an age preoccupied with "perfect babies" (Landsman 2009). This shopper's attitude also emerges among respondents' discussions of high-tech procedures:

> I want twins in my life. That's what I want. Before my sister had had twins I was telling everybody, "I'm about to go to the doctor and stuff like that and have them give me some twins," right? And come to find out twins run in our family. Plus when you get older, it's a high risk of you having twins. It's beautiful. It's a beautiful thing watching them grow. —*LaWanda Jackson, forty-two, African American, single, nursing assistant*

LaWanda does not see multiples as a medical risk—yet they are indeed risky for women and for the babies—but as a desirable product available for a cost. But like any smart shopper, once she realizes that she can get them for free (because of her age and a familial propensity), she decides not to waste her money. The consumer-business dynamic can be less a function of freedom to choose, though, and more about creating needs and reducing human lives and human experiences to commodities.

Adopting Discourses

The commercial talk evaporates when the women contemplate adoption:

> There are a lot of children who need a family. I would do like my mom did, adopt a baby girl. And I say a girl because that's what I want, but if there was a little boy. . . . And it's not like you go to a store and pick and choose, pick and choose, pick and choose. When my mother adopted me, she told me there was a connection. I ran up to her and sat on her lap! —*Nicole Lambert, twenty, African American, single, student*

Adoption involves real children, seen as needy and imperfect, rarely hypothetical designer babies made to reflect parents' good taste. It is tempting to compare the process of selection (e.g., seeking white newborns or attending adoption meet-and-greet events that showcase available children) to shopping. The meant-to-be narrative must be constantly reasserted to deny the commercialization of this aspect of the baby market.

Adoption is salient to infertile and childless women, whether or not they ultimately do it—and most do not. Four of the women I interviewed are adoptive mothers; five are seriously considering it; three tried and failed to adopt; three considered it but rejected the idea (sometimes because their partners demurred); and five might still adopt in the future, but the idea is in the incipient stage. Only a few women choose not to engage with the possibility of adoption. The general attitude in contemporary society is that adoption is a way for almost any woman to become a mother. But the institutions associated with adoption employ a host of screening strategies to funnel in ideal parents and discourage all others, and the process of qualifying is notoriously time consuming and stressful. Despite all this, even more socially marginalized women feel societal pressure to consider adoption and to convincingly account for any decisions not to pursue it in the face of childlessness (there is considerably less pressure to explain forgoing medical treatment).

THE GOOD DEED

> And many times the only time somebody will think of adoption is when they've tried to have their own and can't, and they've exhausted many of the other options or they've just been trying too long and they're tired. Then the heart opens up to, "Maybe I could love someone else's child." —*Annie Adoyo, thirty, second-generation African immigrant, single, student*

Annie mentions to me several times in her interview that adoption might work for her. At one time she says that she thinks of it as her "duty." In the quotation above, she constructs the decision to adopt as not only a last resort for many but also as an awakening of sorts. It is evident in Annie's comments, which both uphold and cast doubt on biologism and ownership, that adoption as a good deed is a complex notion.

Class-based, race-based, and religious subtexts all accompany the narrative of adoption as a good deed. For example, many people tell me that I "did a good thing" in adopting my children or that the children are "lucky" that we adopted them. I usually respond that we parents are the lucky ones to have such wonderful sons. Others—in particular our social workers—see our adoption as guaranteeing the children's upward mobility and as intervening in a cycle of poverty. They are not wrong in this assessment, but attributing all the good fortune to the children (a testament to the social workers' benevolent social engineering) ignores several other outcomes: adoption ended our involuntary childlessness and made us parents; the resulting parent-child relationship is mutually beneficial and satisfying; adoptive parents reap any future rewards of pride, grandchildren, and care in old age; and the birthparents may be deprived of all these benefits. Hannah Johanson's daughter is Chinese, and Hannah and her partner, Gabriel, are white. Strangers see their kinship with their child as up for public discussion, and in well-meaning but offensive ways, these outsiders actively construct the adoption as a good deed:

> Obviously out in society we're encountering lots of questions and comments, which Gabriel and I are still figuring out how to respond to . . . "They don't like little girls in China, do they?" is pretty bad. And I'm glad Jade doesn't understand that yet. —*Hannah Johanson, thirty-nine, white, queer, married, teacher*

This "cross-cutting master narrative of race" (Gailey 2000, 13) is used to portray (white) adoptive parents as rescuing children from an inferior cultural upbringing. In this line of thinking, Chinese girls are saved from Chinese misogyny (and poverty and Communism) and black or Latino children adopted by white parents are protégés being taken on by kind benefactors (Rothman 2005).

The religious subtext of the good-deed model is both prevalent and especially problematic for adoptive parents. Hannah, for example, expresses her annoyance at people who use "her adoption as their political statement" in referring to strangers' approval of what they see as her tacit advocacy of adoption over abortion. In my experience with the mandatory, lengthy adoption-training program provided by the county—and dictated by the state—several of the prospective adoptive parents in the class were looking to adopt because "children need families." For the most part, they were not trying to become parents; they already had children by birth. Instead, adoption is a way to express their (Christian) faith, in some cases, as antiabortionists and as proselytizers. As someone who wanted to adopt to enter motherhood, I could not help but view them as "greedy" competitors for the few available children. Indeed, I was particularly jealous and critical of a woman who worked as a volunteer doula at a Catholic home for "unwed," mostly homeless pregnant women; I felt that she was going to talk a young girl out of keeping the baby she had already been dissuaded from terminating, catch the baby, and then race home with it. But women like these see themselves as morally righteous, and media stories and community feeling support this idea of adoption as a good deed. Many of the women I talked with admire those who could find it in themselves to adopt, but they questioned their own ability to be so selfless and to be tenacious enough to weather the onerous process.

THE IMPOSSIBLE DREAM

The infamously long waiting lists, the intrusive home studies, and apocryphal stories about failed attempts prevent or slow many women—and it is mostly women taking the lead (Rothman 2000b)—from pursuing adoption:

> We even looked into the idea of adoption and later
> on that kind of didn't materialize. I used to work at a
> hospital before, so I knew that there were a lot of babies
> that were born that got adopted or the moms didn't want
> them. And I thought about that, but some of the babies
> were really sick, were drug babies or their mother had
> been an alcoholic or drinking or something that she
> didn't do right in the pregnancy. And so they were called

"drug babies" or whatever, and so those, that's the kind of baby that I wanted to adopt because nobody wanted that child. But somewhere along the line, it didn't happen. I think there was just too many obstacles for us. —*Iris Hernandez, fifty-four, Latina, office assistant*

Whether because of a corrupt bureaucracy or merely because of a less nefarious obstacle course of requirements (made more rigorous for singles and working-class women, and also more legally dicey for lesbians), adoption becomes an unlikely default option for many infertile or involuntarily childless women.

THE INFERIOR CHOICE

Without a doubt, genetic ties and maternal bonding are culturally preferable to adoption. Women are expected to try every way they can to have a biological or genetic child before resorting to adoption (Gailey 2000). Adoption, in this discourse, is an option that (other) people have to settle for when all else fails. The parents' ownership is in question; the kinship ties are thought to be weaker:

> I would love to. But, on the other hand, my husband, he's not as for it as I am. He said he would if I really wanted to, but I don't know if he would love the child any less, but then, that's the one reason why I didn't want to go through with it is because I wouldn't want to put a child into a home where one parent didn't love that child unconditionally like their own. —*Lupe Jimenez, forty-one, Latina, married, electronics technician*

Another concern among the secondarily infertile women I interviewed regards their fear that love and affection would be (unconsciously but inexorably) doled out unevenly between the biological/genetic child and the adopted one. And many of the respondents wonder whether they themselves can muster up enough affection for an adopted child.

Not only is adoption an inferior choice in the hierarchy of procreative options, but many also believe that the children are inferior, that they are damaged in some way or in many ways:

> It's kind of like, if you want a baby, the chances are you're going to get the drug addict baby, and who knows what kind of problems they're going to have. I don't want an older kid because of the issues already. And then I thought maybe I'll go to China or Russia or Poland or whatever. But that's a lot of work. —*Talia Stein, forty-one, white, single, home healthcare aide*

The overblown crack-baby myth (Roberts 1997) and all the real and imagined effects of in utero drug and alcohol exposure feed into the larger social project that constructs adopted children as poor substitutes for hearty and hale, biologically produced, prenatally monitored, properly nurtured, promising middle-class children.

To adopt an infant in the county where I live, the prospective parents must attend not only the standard adoption training but also specialized training about drug-exposed children. Drug exposure is loosely defined as pre- or postnatal illicit drug use (or abuse of legal drugs) by the birth mother or by those who cohabit with her. Jennifer West, a respondent who graduated earlier from the same foster-parent education program I attended, describes the purpose of the training as scare tactics meant to weed out the more cavalier adoptive parents. Class and race come into play as well, of course, with the moral panic about unsuitable prenatal environments directly aimed at poor women and women of color while deflected from higher-status women (who are just as likely to abuse drugs, albeit drugs that are apt to be prescription medications).

In any case, one attitude among infertile and childless women leads to this question: why should stigmatized women be the ones to take stigmatized babies, some of whom require much more care? Women seen as already damaged are asked to adopt babies with more problems than those the average mother has to contend with, and some of the women I interviewed reject this premise. They believe that adoptive kinship ties are not strong enough or permanent enough, and the perceived deficiencies in the children exacerbate this weakness.

THE ETHICALLY QUESTIONABLE

Another way to approach adoption is to question the ethics behind the process. LaWanda Jackson, for example, wonders why a white family would adopt a black child, suggesting that the baby must be some kind of pet or trophy. Her comments reflect a long and ugly legacy of slave children being treated as such by planters' wives and daughters (Rothman 2000b).

Other respondents express concern about the origins of adoptable children, who they suspect—with good cause—might be stolen or given up by coerced birth mothers:

I started researching adoption. I really thought that for a while I was going to do international adoption and adopt from, you know, Central America 'cause I love—I'm really connected with, you know, Central America and Mexico, and I love to speak Spanish. And then I was just researching more, and they were having problems and they had closed down adoption because of—there was some illegal stuff going on. You know, women were being propositioned to sell their babies. So that kind of closed down. *—Jessie Silva, forty-two, white, queer, hair stylist*

Hannah Johanson chose China for her adoption for several reasons. First, she knew that there were orphanages full of baby girls because of the one-child-only policy there and an ancient tradition that favored male heirs. Second, she was worried about getting a child from Eastern Europe because she did not know whether she had the financial resources to provide for an alcohol-exposed or mistreated child that might later exhibit attachment disorder. And, finally, she and her partner, Gabriel, had been told (misled, in my view) that they were unlikely to "qualify" or be chosen for a domestic adoption since they did not own their own home, had only been married a few years, and were not particularly religious. Ethical considerations were also at the forefront of her decision making. In her understanding, the children up for adoption in China were not unloved or necessarily unwanted by their mothers, but they were already detached from them and available.

Transnational adoption of children is a matter for public debate. Conflicts about class, race, national sovereignty, power, and influence came to the fore during the 2006 flap surrounding the white American pop star Madonna's adoption of a black child whose Malawian father was too poor to pay for his care. As a parable about adoption in general, the story exposes several ethical tensions: saving a child versus stealing a child, mothering versus trophy collection, colorblindness versus ethnic/racial preservation.

Despite the caricature of infertile women as tragic figures willing to do anything to get a child, the women I spoke with care very much about the ethical and moral correctness of their child's origins, not least because they will one day have to explain their actions to their child or children.

ADOPTION AGENCY

The women in the interview group who actually did adopt, and the one woman who was herself adopted, offer a more multifaceted picture of adoption:

I felt really angry that I had to do all this to have a child. And here I was this loving, open person with a home and just ready just to give. I was so ready to give but I had to go through this dance. . . . I just got tired. I was just like, "I don't want to stay in this place of anger and it's not going to come to me. A child is not going to come in life." Who would want to come into my life when I feel this way? So I had to change my story around that, too, and I just thought about the child. I just totally got focused and I was like totally open, ready to receive whatever I'm supposed to have—a boy, a girl, you know. Two [years old], an infant. And I'm just going to trust in this process that I'm doing the right thing. So I just got rid of that negative stuff. . . . I can't birth a child, and this is how I'm going to have a child in my life. And this is what feels really real to me. This feels like who I am. To adopt a child feels like more than actually birthing a child. —*Jessie Silva, forty-two, white, queer, hair stylist*

Jessie elevates adoption over birthing a child. She breaks free of her assigned position as a powerless cog squeaking in the wheel of the adoption bureaucracy, a system seemingly designed to cause anxiety. Her shift in mind-set—even finding ways to enjoy the preparations for the arrival of a child as a pregnant women might—represents a departure from the kind of hand-wringing worry that some of the adoptive mothers I spoke with recall and that some of those who consider adoption anticipate. (I experienced such anxiety myself.)

Several of the women take yet another tack that avoids the soul-killing bureaucracy of the adoption process:

I might adopt, but one thing is for sure: I don't have to legally adopt someone to take care of them. I've known a lot of children, and a lot of people who take care of children, and they didn't have to go through the court. You can take a child in, take care of them, clothe them, feed them, and they're someone else's child. I could possibly do that. —*Nicole Lambert, twenty, African American, single, student*

I don't see a problem with adopting or having a foster child. But before I'd adopt or take a foster child, I would take one of my cousins. I have a lot of cousins. Even one of my cousins who is one or two now, by the time I decide to have a child, he would be seven or eight. I would take him, even though I wouldn't have the baby part. . . . My cousin Ursula took in her best friend's daughter. My cousin, the one with the baby, she calls my older cousin Mama. But that's not really her mother. But she took her in, let her stay with her, was helping her with the baby until my cousin got it on her own. Now she's doing it on her own at nineteen. —*Jamilah Washington, nineteen, African American, single, student*

These women refer to the long tradition among African American women of raising other women's children. No home studies, fingerprinting, surprise inspections, court dates, mandatory training, essays, or interviews required. These women bring up a kind of mothering that does not command ownership, "blue-ribbon babies," or perfect blank slates (Gailey 2000). Nor does it mean cutting off birth mothers' rights and privileges. LaWanda Jackson mentions the concept of a "playmom" who mothers a child not hers when the birth mother is unwilling, unavailable, or otherwise unable to do so. These may be long-term or short-term arrangements. Playmoms, godmother aunties, and grandmothers "take on" children, loving them and forming everlasting bonds, all without state approval or state surveillance. These unofficial relationships work well, according to my respondents, until some official document is needed for school, for medical care, or for other agencies. The informal nature of the arrangements also means that they are deprived of the governmental assistance and adoption tax credits that formal adoptive parents receive to ease the financial burden. In most of the United States, efforts are being made to honor so-called kin adoptions and to place forcibly removed children with members of their extended families. But there is a key limitation: in this rule-bound, legal milieu, genetic relationships take precedence over social ones. This expanded approach neglects the fact that a long-time neighbor or dear friend might be much better suited to take in the child than some far-flung relative or a well-meaning but estranged cousin.

Enough Is Enough

Some women find that they do not need to be mothers (or mothers of more than one child) for fulfillment, although this conclusion may be reached only after a woman has traveled some distance toward coming to terms with her childlessness or infertility:

> A couple of women I know have struggled a lot [with childlessness]. One because it was so entrenched in her family. She's Dutch. She said that's just what they do. She didn't feel—she's an incredible artist—so it took her a while to realize that it was okay to give up motherhood for art, and she could be a good enough person in the world. And she battled it for a long time . . . you can tell from her paintings. —*Annette Kramer, fifty-four, white, lesbian, family therapist*

I thought, you know, I don't need a baby to be fulfilled and when I look at my siblings and the responsibility that they have to take on with their children, I think, "Oh I don't think I have it in me to do it. Please call me, I'll come and support you. I'll sit up with you all night." But I just don't think I could do it [on my own]. —*Penny Ortiz, fifty-two, Latina, single, guidance counselor*

Some of the women say that they are already "enough," that, in unselfish ways, they can remain nonmothers (or have only one child) and still contribute to society and be personally satisfied. This attitude contrasts starkly with that of women cited in other studies (originating from treatment populations):

The effect of finding out about the infertility problems for me was that I felt completely useless. I felt like, basically, a piece of garbage. And I thought, "Wait a second, this is not a time for you to feel worthless. This is a time where you really need every ounce of confidence you have." Your feeling of self-worth just plummets when finding this out because everyone always says, "You can have kids. Everyone can have kids. It's the American dream. Why can't you?" "Snap your fingers and you're pregnant!" But if it doesn't work for you . . . I don't even have the words. It just really throws you. (Participant cited by Becker 2000: 39)

It was as if a part of me had died, a part of me was never going to be fulfilled. Grieving to hold a baby. A part of me felt like I was never going to be, a part of me felt like a major disappointment to everybody. (Participant cited by Greil 1991, 54)

We wanted children, and I suppose it's like everybody, you just think it's going to happen . . . and when it doesn't . . . it's devastating. (Participant cited by Franklin 1997, 132)

I got unbearable to live with . . . I was really miserable a lot of the time. You hardly ever saw me with a smile on my face . . . just got really depressed when going through the infertility thing. I used to cry and cry, anything would set me off. (Participant cited by Monach 1993, 112)

It is exceedingly difficult to imagine the women I talked with having such wrenching emotional reactions about their infertility or childlessness. Instead, partly as a result of an ignominious history of exclusion, they cast sidelong glances at the available interventions that would purport to restore a childless or infertile woman to normal by making her a mother. By not trying, they forge an easier path, one that is less crushing.

8

FROM MANDATE TO OPTION

Procreative freedom has to encompass all women to be any freedom at all. To be freely chosen, motherhood and nonmotherhood must be attractive, acceptable options for all women. Fertility monitoring and treatment are not just about women having more choices; these tools are also constantly emerging means for social control. In the interest of true procreative self-determination, it is important to question how we use medicine on women. Sure, the current state of affairs requires advocacy for equitable access to medically assisted reproduction and adoption, but we have to be careful about assuming access is always desirable. And we need to understand that women's real lives ought to shape changes in how these institutions operate.

The simultaneous liberating and oppressing effects of assisted reproduction (and its fallback cousin, adoption) occur on multiple levels. ARTs and the like liberate infertile and involuntarily childless women from "spoiled identity" (Greil 1991): they can become mothers after all and fill the expected role; yet they must admit their failure and submit to sometimes risky, and always rigorous, heavily surveilled medical regimes.

Even the happily childfree come to be viewed as closeted infertiles. Those who do not wish to mother are often treated with disbelief or viewed as slightly pathological when they claim to want a childfree life (Agigian 2008; McQuillan et al. 2011;

Morell 2000). Single women and lesbians can become mothers without men as partners—but they usually must trade one form of patriarchy for another as doctors, psychologists, social workers, intimates, colleagues, and even casual bystanders scrutinize their fitness for motherhood. At the same time that motherhood is opened up to more women, the notion of motherhood as the pinnacle of womanhood regains strength.

Assisted reproduction and adoption help normalize those women who cannot become mothers in the conventional way. Women from all backgrounds are generally expected to address their infertility or childlessness despite systematic barriers to the available interventions. And many of these same women tout the motherhood mandate for others while exempting themselves on the basis of what they see as their intrinsic difference from most women.

These options that ameliorate infertility or childlessness for some women also, at the same time, challenge essentialist ideas about motherhood as a whole. The assumption of motherhood as sacred, natural, normal—and biological and genetic—gets destabilized. However, codifying familial relationships and kinships, a continuing legal maneuver in the light of the complex relationships engendered by medically assisted conception, sometimes ends up denying integral social relationships. The kinds of informal mothering arrangements practiced most often in minority communities represent a mode of resistance to dominant meanings of womanhood, motherhood, infertility, childlessness, and family. These need to be recognized and allowed by schools, medical authorities, and the legal system. The disruption by ART of the historic linearity in kin relationships (though originating among the white middle class) can actually help by contributing new imaginings of relatedness (Strathern 1992).

Fertility clinics and providers extol the ethical and business-growing benefits of serving singles and lesbians. Yet, predicated on legal risks, a fear of HIV, the value-added quality (read: eugenics) of ARTs, and a cultural turn toward greater medical control of women's bodies, the once-empowering turkey basters are being left to Thanksgiving duties in favor of the expert's syringe and powerful medications. Increased choices can lead to increased control in some respects and also, unfortunately, to the dangers of treatments gone awry (hyperstimulated ovaries and births of multiples are not rare and the increased risk of breast cancer and ovarian cancer—though purposefully downplayed by fertility consultants—is particularly worrisome).

Adoption has the potential to liberate, to create transfamilies. Transnational, transracial, multilingual, multicultural, two-mother, two-father, and queer families are more common than ever before (Child Welfare Gateway 2008). Adoption transforms the meaning of families by changing the way families look and the way family gets experienced. Motherhood and parenthood in general are set free from biologic and genetic roots, from pregnancy and childbirth, from looking like one's young, even from beginning mothering at the child's infancy. The need to mother supplants the need for following the traditional, linear route to motherhood. A childless woman is normalized as a mother (read: a true woman) through adoption at the same time that her actions expand the definitions and discourses of motherhood and mothering (Park 2006). But the displacement—some say "trafficking"—of children preferably, for many, involves matching race and the selection of only the youngest, healthiest children for assimilation into a now-"normal" family. Happy families are created, to be sure, but the distinct preference and unsatisfied demand for particular children further oppresses those for whom this type of motherhood is denied—to say nothing of the thousands of children who remain left out.

More adopters, numerically speaking, are not desirable since adoption cannot be a long-term feminist solution to infertility or involuntary childlessness, as Barbara Katz Rothman (2005) persuasively argues. For poor women to lose their children through state intervention or to feel compelled to "choose" to give them up in the face of economic circumstance and its consequences (e.g., inadequately treated drug addiction) is not the natural order of things: it is the result of a failure on the part of society to equitably distribute resources. Still, women from working-class backgrounds and women who are ethnic or racial minorities might find adoption a more interesting prospect if the process was affirming instead of alienating.

Stratified reproduction (Ginsburg and Rapp 1995) notwithstanding, opportunities for unconventional routes to motherhood and mothering are increasing for socially marginalized women (Culley et al. 2009; Greil 2009; Inhorn et al. 2009). Public health advocacy by fertility clinicians and social researchers concerned about disparities in access to fertility treatment, media stories about miracle babies, mandatory insurance coverage pushed through by legislators in some states, and clinics' need for new markets have all resulted in greater use of these services by women other than the white, middle-class married women for whom the procedures were originally intended. Some (e.g., Thompson 2002) suggest that formal barriers no longer exist to any significant degree for single women and lesbians. But poor and working-class African American, Latino, and Arab American infertile couples (in a study of *married* infertile people) are routinely denied sufficient insurance, savings, and adequate information to access treatment (Inhorn et al. 2009). Cultural and religious factors also impede some ethnic minorities from making use of donor gametes or from adopting outside their families. The resulting disparities vex social-justice-minded researchers in light of the fact that these are the very groups most likely to be medically infertile.

Disrupted Definitions:
Recasting Infertility and Childlessness

Infertility and involuntary childlessness do not always spell a life crisis. As researchers, we ask women when they discovered their infertility, how they coped, and how others reacted (e.g., see appendixes of Becker 2000; Greil 1991; Harwood 2007; Szkupinski-Quiroga 2002). My respondents' blank stares at these inquiries gave me pause. It became clear that *my* life crisis was not theirs. I slowly realized that childlessness or infertility could be a gradual process with meanings different from my own and could have unexpected potential for quasi emancipation from predominant notions of motherhood. These women's perspectives and experiences make it clear that infertility and childlessness do not have to be a predicament. Just as motherhood is not necessarily a *chosen* role and does not always equate to fulfillment, infertility and childlessness are often not chosen, but they do not preclude fulfillment.

Most of the study respondents do not recall a traumatic moment of hearing an infertility diagnosis or recognizing their permanent childlessness. Their suffering over their "disrupted reproduction" is mild compared to that reported in most other ethnographic works. Their stances are decidedly ambivalent, be they de facto infertile, infertile identified, or childfree by choice, or whether childlessness "just happened" or whether they have intentionally delayed childbearing. As a whole, they are not particularly regretful in retrospect; they emphasize the many positive aspects to not having children or to having only one.

The women's comments and reasoning demonstrate a familiarity with the master cultural narratives about infertile and childless women and about motherhood and mothering. Their lived realities do not match the cultural discourse (this finding parallels Becky Thompson's (1994) study of African American women with eating disorders in a society where this is thought to be a white girl's problem). The women I talked with accommodate the popular points of view but resist the inherent constraints. The women of *Not Trying* approach medically assisted procreation and adoption in deliberate, defiant ways. Azra scoffs at her doctors' suggestion that "stress" impacts her fertility; Penny becomes outraged at a doctor who tries to sell her on fertility treatment; Jamilah disbelieves in the biological clock as she witnesses her relatives in their forties having babies; and Dianne takes charge of her surgical procedure. Although several discussed medical treatment as something that other, more privileged women who trust doctors might invest in, they note that they themselves do not need a man to become pregnant (there are sperm banks, after all) and that opportunities for unofficial adoption are not rare. Jessie and Jennifer both forge ahead with the trying bureaucratic process of adoption, creating meant-to-be personal myths and choosing to ignore warnings and "scare tactics" from social workers trying to prepare them for possible disappointment.

The women consistently deny labels like "intentionally child-free" (Karen wonders how she ended up childless, but it is not something she ever thinks much about) and "infertile," something that only has meaning to those on the road to treatment (even the postmenopausal respondents and Zara, whose uterus is severely damaged, will not accept this designation). Ambivalence about one's infertility was acceptable before the technological cures came on the scene (Earle and Letherby 2007. A respondent in one study says that she never felt desperate about having a baby until she got involved in IVF treatment, at which point she became so invested in the goal that when it did not work, she felt something was taken away from her (Franklin 1997, 182). Survey data also show that being in treatment is positively correlated with identifying as infertile (Johnson and

Fledderjohann 2012). This phenomenon partly accounts for my respondents' acceptance of their childlessness. Rather than the desperate infertile (a category that actually describes few infertile women), many of my respondents could be called the "pragmatic infertile."

Those whom I describe as "infertile identified" are precisely the ones willing to explore adoption or try some of the medical techniques available (within reason), but many of the others, those who do not accept the infertile label, do not go that far. The available terms cannot begin to explain their nonmotherhood status. Many of my respondents pay lip service to the rhetoric of desperation and loss of femininity even while exercising their personal agency by either declining treatment or adoption or by pursuing (or imagining pursuing) either on their own terms. As when they dismiss the idea of adoption but feel compelled to carefully explain this choice or when they put off decision-making about motherhood, they resist medical and bureaucratic control while still pointing out that the mere existence of assisted reproduction and adoption has relevance to their own lives.

Any frustration about lack of access to treatment or insufficient capital to cover adoption takes a backseat to other pragmatic (yet shifting) concerns like readiness for motherhood, locating a suitable life partner, and coping with other life events. At the same time, they piously (or, in many cases, matter of factly) accept God's—or the universe's—preordained plan for them to become mothers or not. Coupled with distrust of medicalization and adoption, they maintain a come-what-may attitude instead of relentlessly pursuing motherhood.

They do not report much angst, but the women still have deep feelings about it all. The childfree express some sadness at times, and the involuntarily childless or secondarily infertile tend to temper any regret with optimism about their present and future circumstances.

While it is true that the study participants were the ones who were willing to talk about experiences that are painful to some women, this self-selection bias does not detract from the fact that their experiences are important, too. Their life experiences underscore the possibility that infertility and childlessness need not be tragic. Ambivalence better describes women's real experience with infertility and involuntary childlessness. At times they regret; at times they feel fulfilled.

By extension, and though we work to disguise it, motherhood and voluntary childlessness are also fraught with ambivalence. The lesson is that women's real experiences do not easily fit into our preexisting categories (see also Greil and McQuillan 2010). Fertile or infertile, voluntarily or involuntarily childless, these definitions contract and expand depending on who uses them and when and where along the life-course experience a woman may be.

A first step toward a more holistic vision of infertility and childlessness involves dismantling the accepted notions that the infertile are probably involuntarily childless and that any woman who is childfree either chose her status or is sad if she did not choose it. More work is needed to understand how childless women from diverse backgrounds make meaning of their circumstances, given their different social histories and contemporary positions in the social hierarchy.

Factors like class, sexual identity, marital status, culture, region, age, and able-bodiedness clearly matter a great deal as the experiences of the women I interviewed suggest. Additional research would likely help us understand how these statuses interact in infertile and childless women's lives. We also know little about the views of women with disabilities whose rights and access to motherhood is delegitimized because of ableism. Inhorn et al. (2009, 187) mention that childless Latinas fear that the use of the term "infertile" will curse them and that infertile African Americans see ARTs as a "white thing." One is left to wonder whether infertility as a concept only applies to white, middle- and upper-class, able-bodied, straight women. It may be a clandestine identity for some other women, or they may see it as a privileged status to which they do not have access. What is more, the meaning of infertility may well change among new cohorts coming of age after treatment has become more successful and routinized.

One way to interrogate the commonalities and differences among women would be to conduct focus groups with treatment seekers and nonseekers who could share their rationale and perhaps reveal what makes them head in opposite directions.

Interviewing women who are more militantly childfree alongside ambivalent nonmothers, unintentional mothers, and intentional mothers may be a way to capture a fuller range of women's experience. It is also important to examine more closely the motivations and insights of medical workers involved in fertility treatment as well as those of adoption social workers if we are to understand how they help shape the experience for women. It is worth exploring the ways in which widespread medicalization and acceptance of ARTs impacts women's beliefs about kinship, eugenics, and the life course, whether they use the technologies or not.

Current trends in hyperintensive mothering based on attachment theory—in which women are told that motherhood par excellence entails babywearing (into late toddlerhood), cobathing, cosleeping, and extended breastfeeding as well as providing play dates, enrichment classes, and appropriate developmental toys—has to play into the optionality of motherhood. Further research could clarify the relationship between these ideas.

There is still plenty of unexplained variance for disparate interest in seeking help with fertility (Greil 2009). Quantitative testing of theoretical concepts like "ambivalent childlessness" may elucidate persistent questions about marginalized women's help seeking. Expense and recruitment challenges aside, longitudinal studies of changing feelings and attitudes about infertility are sorely needed. How do the formerly infertile or involuntarily childless (or, for that matter, the once adamantly childfree) feel years later, when their status is resolved or remains unchanged?

Women should not be made to feel that motherhood (or the pursuit of motherhood) must define them—or that childlessness or infertility must mark them as deviant. I hope that the category-defying experiences and the thoughtful words of the women who participated in my research will help scholars rethink customary approaches to the study of infertility and childlessness and to problematize the dichotomies of motherhood versus nonmotherhood and involuntary versus voluntary childlessness. The stories of the women I talked with provoke a rethinking of theories about women's decisionmaking and attitudes about treatment and adoption in the United States.

Concerns about access disparities are important, but it is equally vital to expand what womanhood and fulfillment mean. Medicalization is a powerful normalizing institution that can challenge women's procreative liberty. It is the task of feminists to chip away at the uneven distribution of power. Marginalized women—in a sense, the original feminists—provide some likely tools.

APPENDIX

All names used in this book are pseudonyms, a few chosen by the respondents themselves; I attempt to preserve the ethnic origin suggested by their actual names. All the women listed as infertile are either medically or personally identified as such; but that identification occurs along a spectrum, and none are "definitely" infertile, according to them. For women with no knowledge of their fertility, I indicate their childlessness, their menopausal status, or both. I include occupation as an imperfect proxy for class; the benefit of using occupation is that the category taps into common notions of prestige. Fifteen of the participants could be considered "working class"; the rest qualify as "middle class." I use the term "queer" for sexual minorities who choose to identify that way. The race/ethnicity descriptions also reflect their self-reports; two (Zara Senai and Azra Alic) are naturalized citizens, and the rest are US born. "Secondary infertility" means that the woman has at least one child, wants or wanted more, but cannot have them biologically for medical reasons.

Identifier	Age	Race/ethnicity	Sexual Identity	Marital Status	Occupation	Fertility/Motherhood Status
Annie Adoyo	30	Kenyan	Straight	Single	Student	Childless
Azra Alic	30	Bosnian	Straight	Partnered	Apartment manager	IVF patient
Mary Benson	48	African American	Straight	Married	Cook	Infertile/childless
Lourdes Garcia	56	Latina	Unsure	Single	Administrative assistant	Childless
Iris Hernandez	54	Latina	Straight	Partnered	Administrative assistant	Infertile/childless
LaWanda Jackson	42	African American	Straight	Single	Nursing assistant	Infertile/childless
Dianne Jacobsen	58	White	Straight	Single	Life coach	Infertile/adoptive mother
Lupe Jimenez	41	Latina	Straight	Married	Pharmacy technician	Secondary infertility
Hannah Johanson	39	White	Queer	Married	Teacher	Infertile/adoptive mother
Shana Jones	25	African American	Straight	Single	Student	Childless
Annette Kramer	54	White	Lesbian	Partnered	Nurse	Childless
Nicole Lambert	20	African American	Straight	Single	Student	Childless
Serena Lopez	39	Latina	Straight	Married	Laboratory technician	Secondary infertility
Lana Marks	52	White	Lesbian	Partnered	Therapist	Childless
Aikiko Moto	43	Japanese American	Straight	Married	Teacher	Secondary infertility
Penny Ortiz	52	Latina	Straight	Single	Guidance counselor	Postmenopausal/childless
Gloria Owusu	38	Ghanaian	Straight	Single	Project manager	Childless
Carol P.	50s	White	Straight	Married	Fertility counselor	n/a—expert
Emily Reilly	30	White	Straight	Single	Fast food manager	Childless
Zara Senai	45	Somalian	Straight	Married	Laboratory technician	Infertile/childless
Jessie Silva	42	Portuguese	Queer	Single	Hairstylist	Infertile/adoptive mother
Robin Smith	42	White	Lesbian	Partnered	Fertility counselor	IVF patient
Talia Stein	41	Israeli	Straight	Single	Home health care aide	Childless
Karen Tabb	49	White	Straight	Single	Teacher	Postmenopausal/childless
Jamilah Washington	19	African American	Straight	Single	Student	Childless
Jennifer West	46	Latina	Straight	Married	Civil engineer	Infertile/adoptive mother

REFERENCES

Abbey, Antonia, Frank M. Andrews, and L. Jill Halman. 1992. "Infertility and Subjective Well-Being: The Mediating Roles of Self-Esteem, Internal Control, and Interpersonal Conflict." *Journal of Marriage and Family* 54 (2): 408–17.

Abma, Joyce C., and Gladys M. Martinez. 2006. "Childlessness among Older Women in the United States: Trends And Profiles." *Journal of Marriage and the Family* 68 (4): 1045–56.

Agigian, Amy. 2004. *Baby Steps: How Lesbian Alternative Insemination Is Changing the World.* Middlebury, CT: Wesleyan University Press.

Alexander, Baine, Robert Rubenstein, Marcene Goodman, and Mark Luborsky. 1992. "A Path Not Taken: A Cultural Analysis of Regrets and Childlessness in the Lives of Older Women." *Gerontologist* 32 (5): 618–26.

Alexander, Michelle. 2012. *The New Jim Crow: Mass Incarceration in the Age of Colorblindness.* New York: New Press.

Allison, Jill. 2011. "Conceiving Silence: Infertility as Discursive Contradiction in Ireland." *Medical Anthropology Quarterly* 25 (1): 1–21.

Anderson, Elijah. 1999. *Code of the Street: Decency, Violence, and the Moral Life of the Inner City.* New York: W. W. Norton.

Associated Press. 2007. "India's Surrogate Mother Business Raises Questions of Global Ethics." *New York Daily News*, December 30. *www.nydailynews.com/news/world/india-surrogate-mother-business-raises-questions-global-ethics-article-1.276982#ixzz2qgh2zB5P.*

Barrett, Geraldine, and Kaye Wellings. 2002. "What Is a 'Planned' Pregnancy? Empirical Data From a British Study." *Social Science and Medicine* 55 (4): 545–57.

Becker, Gaylene. 2000. *The Elusive Embryo: How Women and Men Approach New Reproductive Technologies.* Berkeley: University of California Press.

Bell, Ann V. 2009. "'It's Way Out of My League': Low-Income Women's Experiences of Medicalized Infertility." *Gender and Society* 23 (5): 688–709.

Bell, Ann V. 2010. "Beyond (Financial) Accessibility: Inequalities within the Medicalisation of Infertility." *Sociology of Health and Illness* 32 (4): 631–46.

Britt, Elizabeth C. 2001. *Conceiving Normalcy: Law, Rhetoric, and the Double Binds of Infertility.* Tuscaloosa: University of Alabama Press.

Bulcroft, Richard, and Jay Teachman. 2004. "Ambiguous Constructions: Development of a Childless or Childfree Life Course." In *Handbook of Contemporary Families,* edited by M. Coleman and L. H. Ganong, 114–35. Newbury Park, CA: Sage.

Bureau of Consular Affairs. 2008. "Statistics: Immigrant Visas Issued to Orphans Coming to the United States." Washington, DC: US Department of State. *www.travel.state.gov/family/adoptions/stats/stats451.html.*

Carmichael, Gordon A., and Andrea Whittaker. 2007. "Choice and Circumstance: Qualitative Insights into Contemporary Childlessness in Australia." *European Journal of Population–Revue Europeene De Demographie* 23: 111–43.

Casper, Monica. 1998. *The Making of the Unborn Patient: A Social Anatomy of Fetal Surgery.* New Brunswick, NJ: Rutgers University Press.

Centers for Disease Control and Prevention (CDC). 1983. *Surgical Sterilization and Surveillance: Tubal Sterilization and Hysterectomy in Women Aged 15–44, Summary 1979–1980.* Atlanta: CDC.

———. 1997. *Fertility, Family Planning, and Women's Health: New Data from the 1995 National Survey of Family Growth. Centers for Disease Control and Prevention, US Department of Health and Human Services.* Atlanta: CDC.

———. 2004. *Health, United States 2003.* National Center for Health Statistics. Atlanta: CDC.

———. 2009. "National Survey of Family Growth 2006." *www.cdc.gov/nchs/nsfg/nsfg_2006_2010_puf.htm.*

————. 2012. "National Survey of Family Growth 2006–2010." *www.cdc.gov/nchs/nsfg/key_statistics/i.htm#infertility.*

Child Welfare Information Gateway. 2008. "Adoption." *www.childwelfare.gov/adoption.*

Chodorow, Nancy. 1978. *The Reproduction of Mothering: Psychoanalysis and the Sociology of Gender.* Berkeley: University of California Press.

Clarke, Adele. 1998. *Disciplining Reproduction: Modernity, American Life Sciences, and "The Problems of Sex."* Berkeley: University of California Press.

Collins, Patricia Hill. 1991. *Black Feminist Thought: Knowledge, Consciousness, and the Politics of Empowerment.* New York: Routledge.

————. 1999. "Will the Real Mother Please Stand Up? The Logic of Eugenics and American National Family Planning." In *Revisioning Women, Health, and Healing: Feminist Cultural, and Technoscience Perspectives,* edited by Adele E. Clarke and Virginia Olesen, 266–82. New York: Routledge.

Crowe, Christine. 1985. "'Women Want It': *In Vitro* Fertilization and Women's Motivations for Participation." *Women's Studies International Forum* 8 (6): 547–52.

Culley, Lorraine. 2009. "Dominant Narratives and Excluded Voices: Research on Ethnic Differences in Access to Assisted Conception in More Developed Societies." In Culley et al. 2009, 17–33.

Culley, Lorraine, Nicky Hudson, and Floor Van Roolj, eds. 2009. *Marginalized Reproduction: Ethnicity, Infertility, and Reproductive Technologies.* London: Earthscan.

Davis, Angela. 1981. *Women, Race, and Class.* New York: Random House.

————. 1998. "Surrogates and Outcast Mothers: Racism and Reproductive Politics in the Nineties." In *The Angela Davis Reader,* edited by Joy James, 210–21. Malden, MA: Blackwell.

Dodge, Mary, and Gilbert Geis. 2003. *Stealing Dreams: A Fertility Clinic Scandal.* Boston: Northeastern University Press.

Dorow, Sara K. 2006. *Transnational Adoption: A Cultural Economy of Race, Gender, and Kinship.* New York: New York University Press.

Duncan, Simon, and Birgit Pfau-Effinger. 2000. *Gender, Economy, and Culture in the European Union.* New York: Routledge.

Duster, Troy. 2003. *Backdoor to Eugenics.* 2nd ed. New York: Routledge.

Dworkin, Andrea. 1983. *Right-Wing Women.* New York: Perigee Books.

Earle, Sarah, and Gayle Letherby. 2007. "Conceiving Time? Women Who Do or Do Not Conceive." *Sociology of Health and Illness* 29 (2): 233–50. Edin, Kathryn, and Maria Kefalas. 2005. *Promises I Can Keep: Why Poor Women Put Motherhood Before Marriage.* Berkeley: University of California Press.

Ettore, Elizabeth. 2002. *Reproductive Genetics, Gender, and the Body.* New York: Routledge.

Everingham, Christine. 1994. *Motherhood and Modernity: An Investigation into the Rational Dimension of Mothering.* Buckingham, PA: Open University Press.

Exley, Catherine, and Gayle Letherby. 2001. "Managing a Disrupted Lifecourse: Issues of Identity and Emotion Work." *Health: An Interdisciplinary Journal for the Social Study of Health, Illness and Medicine* 5 (1): 112–32.

Ferre Institute. 2001. "The Hidden Problem of Infertility in the African American Community." *www.ferre.org/foci/hidden.html.*

Fessler, Ann. 2006. *The Girls Who Went Away: The Hidden History of the Women who Surrendered Children for Adoption in the Decades before Roe v. Wade.* New York: Penguin Press.

Firestone, Shulamith. 1970. *The Dialectic of Sex: The Case for Feminist Revolution.* New York: Morrow.

Fisher, Allen P. 2003. "Still 'Not Quite as Good as Having Your Own?' Toward a Sociology of Adoption." *Annual Review of Sociology* 29: 335–61.

Franklin, Sarah. 1997. *Embodied Progress: A Cultural Account of Assisted Conception.* New York: Routledge.

Gailey, Christine Ward. 2000. "Ideologies of Motherhood and Kinship in US Adoption." In *Ideologies of Motherhood: Race, Class, Sexuality,*

Nationalism, edited by Helena Ragone and France Winddance Twine, 11–55. New York: Routledge.

Gillespie, Rosemary. 2000. "When No Means No: Disbelief, Disregard, and Deviance as Discourses of Voluntary Childlessness." *Women's Studies International Forum* 23 (2): 223–34.

Ginsburg, Faye. 1989. *Contested Lives: The Abortion Debate in an American Community.* Berkeley: University of California Press.

Ginsburg, Faye, and Rayna Rapp, eds. 1995. *Conceiving the New World Order: The Global Politics of Reproduction.* Berkeley: University of California Press.

Goffman, Erving. 1963. *Stigma: Notes on the Management of Spoiled Identity.* New York: Simon and Schuster.

Gregory, Elizabeth. 2007. *Ready: Why Women are Embracing the New Late Motherhood.* Philadelphia: Basic Books.

Greil, Arthur L. 1997. "Infertility and Psychological Distress: A Critical Review of the Literature." *Social Science and Medicine* 45 (11): 1679–784.

———. 1991. *Not Yet Pregnant: Infertile Couples in Contemporary America.* New Brunswick, NJ: Rutgers University Press.

Greil, Arthur L., and Julia McQuillan. 2010. "'Trying' Times: Medicalization, Intent, and Ambiguity in the Definition of Infertility." *Medical Anthropology Quarterly* 24 (3): 137–52.

Greil, Arthur L., Julia McQuillan, Katherine M. Johnson, Kathleen S. Slauson-Blevins, and Karina M. Shreffler. 2009. "The Hidden Infertile: Infertile Women without Pregnancy Intent in the United States." *Fertility and Sterility* 93 (6): 2080–83.

Greil, Arthur L., Julia McQuillan, and Kathleen S. Slauson-Blevins. 2011. "The Social Construction of Infertility." *Social Compass* 5 (8): 736–46.

Greil, Arthur L., Julia McQuillan, Karina M. Shreffler, Katherine M. Johnson, and Kathleen S. Slauson-Blevins. 2011. "Race/Ethnicity and Medical Services for Infertility: Stratified Reproduction in a

Population-Based Sample of U.S. Women." *Journal of Health and Social Behavior* 52 (4): 493–507.

Greil, Arthur L., Karina M. Shreffler, Lone Schmidt, and Julia McQuillan. 2011. "Variation in Distress Among Infertile Women: Evidence from a Population-Based Sample." *Human Reproduction* 14 (8): 2101–12.

Habermas, Jürgen. 1990. *Moral Consciousness and Communicative Action.* Translated by Christian Lenhardt and Shierry Weber Nicholsen. Cambridge, MA: MIT Press.

Handwerker, Lisa. 2000. "The Politics of Making Modern Babies in China: Reproductive Politics and the 'New' Eugenics." In *Ideologies and Technologies of Motherhood: Race, Class, Sexuality, and Nationalism,* edited by Helena Ragone and France Winddance Twine, 298–333. New York: Routledge.

Haraway, Donna. 1991. *Simians, Cyborgs, and Women: The Reinvention of Nature.* New York: Routledge.

Hartsock, Nancy C. M. 1983. *Money, Sex, and Power: Toward a Feminist Historical Materialism.* New York: Longman.

Harwood, Karey. 2007. *The Infertility Treadmill: Feminist Ethics, Personal Choice, and the Use of Reproductive Technologies.* Chapel Hill: University of North Carolina Press.

Hays, Sharon. 1998. *The Cultural Contradictions of Motherhood.* New Haven, CT: Yale University Press.

Haynes, Jane, and Juliet Miller. 2003. *Inconceivable Conceptions: Psychological Aspects of Infertility and Reproductive Technology.* New York: Routledge.

Houseknecht, Sharon. 1987. "Voluntary Childlessness." *Handbook of Marriage and the Family,* edited by Marvin B. Sussman and Suzanne K. Steinmetz, 384–93. New York: Plenum Press.

Inhorn, Marcia C. 2000. "Missing Motherhood: Infertility, Technology, and Poverty in Egyptian Women's Lives." In *Ideologies and Technologies of Motherhood: Race, Class, Sexuality, and Nationalism,* edited by Helena Ragone and France Winddance Twine, 139–68. New York: Routledge.

Inhorn, Marcia, Rosario Ceballo, and Robert Natchigall. 2009. "Marginalized, Invisible, and Unwanted: American Minority Struggles with Infertility and Assisted Conception." In Culley et al. 2009, 181–98. London: Earthscan.

Inhorn, Marcia, ed. 2007. *Reproductive Disruptions: Gender, Technology and Biopolitics in the New Millennium.* New York: Berghahn Books.

InterNational Council for Infertility Information Dissemination (INCIID). *www.inciid.org.*

Jacobson, Heather. 2008. *Culture Keeping: White Mothers, International Adoption, and the Negotiation of Family Difference.* Nashville: Vanderbilt University Press.

Jeffries, Sherryl, and Candace Konnert, C. 2002. "Regret and Psychological Well-Being among Voluntarily and Involuntarily Childless Women and Mothers." *International Journal on Aging and Human Development* 54 (2): 89–102.

Johnson, Katherine. 2009. "The (Single) Woman Question: Ideological Barriers to Accessing Fertility Treatment." Paper presented in August at the annual meeting of the Society for the Study of Social Problems, San Francisco.

Johnson, Katherine, and Jasmine Fledderjohann. 2012. "Revisiting 'Her' Infertility: Medicalized Embodiment, Self-Identification and Distress." *Social Science and Medicine* 75 (5): 883–91.

Kemkes-Grottenthaler, Ariane. 2003. "Postponing or Rejecting Motherhood: Results of a Survey among Female Academic Professionals." *Journal of Biosocial Science* 35 (2): 213–26.

Kirkman, Maggie. 2001. "Thinking of Something to Say: Public and Private Narratives of Infertility." *Health Care for Women International* 22 (6): 523–35.

Klein, Renate, and Robyn Rowland. 1989. "Hormone Cocktails: Women as Test-Sites for Fertility Drugs." *Women's Studies International Forum* 12 (1): 333–48.

Kneale, Dylan, and Heather Joshi. 2008. "Postponement and Childlessness: Evidence from Two British Cohorts." *Demographic Research* 19: 1935–64.

Klett-Davies, Martina. 2007. *Going it Alone? Lone Motherhood in Late Modernity*. Hampshire, UK: Ashgate.

Koropeckyj-Cox, Tanya. 2002. "Beyond Parental Status: Psychological Well-Being in Middle and Old Age." *Journal of Marriage and Family* 64 (4): 957–71.

Koropeckyj-Cox, Tanya, Amy M. Pienta, and Tyson H. Brown. 2007. "Women of the 1950s and the 'Normative' Life Course: The Implications of Childlessness, Fertility Timing, and Marital Status for Psychological Well-Being in Late Midlife." *International Journal of Aging and Human Development* 64 (4): 299–330.

Koropeckyj-Cox, Tanya, Victor Romano, and Amanda Moras. 2007. "Through the Lenses of Gender, Race, and Class: Students' Perceptions of Childless/Childfree Individuals and Couples." *Sex Roles* 56 (7–8): 415–28.

Ladd-Taylor, Molly, and Lauri Umansky. 1998. *"Bad Mothers": The Politics of Blame in Twentieth Century America*. New York: New York University Press.

Landsman, Gail. 2009. *Reconstructing Motherhood and Disability in an Age of "Perfect" Babies*. New York: Routledge.

Lasker, Judith, and Susan Borg. 1994. *In Search of Parenthood: Coping with Infertility and High-Tech Conception*. Philadelphia: Temple University Press.

Letourneau, Rene, ed. 2012. "Global Infertility Drugs, Devices Market to Approach $4.8B in 2017." *Healthcare Finance News*, October 3. *www.healthcarefinancenews.com/news/global-infertility-drugs-devices-market-approach-48b-2017*.

Letherby, Gayle. 1999. "Other than Mother and Mothers as Others: The Experience of Motherhood and Non-Motherhood in Relation to 'Infertility' and 'Involuntary Childlessness.'" *Women's Studies International Forum* 22 (3): 359–72.

———. 2002a. "Challenging Dominant Discourses: Identity and Change and the Experience of 'Infertility' and 'Involuntary Childlessness.'" *Journal of Gender Studies* 11 (3): 277–88.

———. 2002b. "Childless and Bereft? Stereotypes and Realities in Relation to 'Voluntary' and 'Involuntary' Childlessness and Womanhood." *Sociological Inquiry* 72 (1): 7–20.

Lewin, Ellen. 1993. *Lesbian Mothers: Accounts of Gender in American Culture.* Ithaca, NY: Cornell University Press.

Livingston, Gretchen, and D'vera Cohn. 2010. *Childlessness Up among All Women; Down among Women with Advanced Degrees.* Washington, DC: Pew Research Center.

Lock, Margaret. 2007. "The Final Disruption? Biopolitics of Post-Reproductive Life." In *Reproductive Disruptions: Gender, Technology, and Biopolitics in the New Millennium,* edited by Marcia C. Inhorn, 200–24. New York: Berghahn Books.

Lombardo, Marina. 2009. "Emotionally Speaking." *Conceive Magazine,* February, 30–33.

Mamo, Laura. 2007. *Queering Reproduction: Achieving Pregnancy in the Age of Technoscience.* Durham, NC: Duke University Press.

Marsh, Margaret S., and Wanda Ronner. 1996. *The Empty Cradle: Infertility in America from Colonial Times to Present.* Baltimore: Johns Hopkins University Press.

———. 2008. *The Fertility Doctor: John Rock and the Reproduction Revolution.* Baltimore: Johns Hopkins University Press.

Martin, Emily. 1987. *The Woman in the Body: A Cultural Analysis of Reproduction.* Boston: Beacon Press.

Matthews, Ralph, and Anne Martin Matthews. 1986. "Infertility and Involuntary Childlessness: The Transition to Non-parenthood." *Journal of Marriage and Family* 48 (3): 641–49.

Matthews, Sandra, and Laura Wexler. 2000. *Pregnant Pictures.* New York: Routledge.

May, Elaine Tyler. 1995. *Barren in the Promised Land: Childless Americans and the Pursuit of Happiness.* New York: Basic Books.

McQuillan, Julia, Arthur L. Greil, Karina M. Shreffler, Patricia A. Wonch-Hill, Kari C. Gentzler, and John D. Hathcoat. 2012. "Does the Reason Matter? Childlessness Concerns among U.S. Women." *Journal of Marriage and Family* 74 (5): 1166–81.

McQuillan, Julia, Arthur L. Greil, Lynn White, and Mary Casey Jacob. 2003. "Frustrated Fertility: Infertility and Psychological Distress among Women." *Journal of Marriage and Family* 65 (4): 1007–19.

McQuillan, Julia, Arthur L. Greil, and Karina M. Shreffler. 2011. "Pregnancy Intentions of Those Who Do Not Try: Focusing On Women Who Are Okay Either Way." *Maternal and Child Health Journal* 15 (2): 178–87.

Miall, Charlene. 1994. "Community Constructs of Involuntary Childlessness: Sympathy, Stigma, and Social Support." *Canadian Review of Sociology and Anthropology* 31 (4): 392–422.

Mies, Maria. 1987. "Sexist and Racist Implications of New Reproductive Technologies." *Alternatives* 12 (3): 323–42.

Monach, James. 1993. *Childless, No Choice: The Experience of Involuntary Childlessness.* New York: Routledge.

Moore, Lisa Jean. 2007. *Sperm Counts: Overcome by Man's Most Precious Fluid.* New York: New York University Press.

Moos, Merry K., Ruth Petersen, Katherine Meadows, Cathy L. Melvin, and Alison M. Spitz. 1997. "Pregnant Women's Perspectives on Intendedness of Pregnancy." *Women's Health Issues* 7 (6): 385–92.

Morgan, Lynn. 2006. "Strange Anatomy: Gertrude Stein and the Avant-Garde Embryo." *Hypatia* 21 (1): 15–34.

Morgan, Lynn M., and Meredith W. Michaels, eds. 1999. *Fetal Subjects, Feminist Positions.* Philadelphia: University of Pennsylvania Press.

Moynihan, Daniel Patrick. 1965. *The Negro Family: The Case for National Action.* Washington, DC: US Department of Labor.

Mundy, Liza. 2007. *Everything Conceivable: How Assisted Reproduction is Changing Men, Women, and the World.* New York: Alfred A. Knopf.

National Association of Black Social Workers. Reports available from *www.nabsw.org.*

Nelson, Jennifer. 2003. *Women of Color and the Reproductive Rights Movement.* New York: New York University Press.

Nsiah-Jefferson, Laurie, and Elaine J. Hall. 1989. "Reproductive Technology: Perspectives and Implications for Low-Income Women and Women of Color." In *Healing Technology: Feminist Perspectives,* edited by Kathryn Strother Ratcliff, 93–118. Ann Arbor: University of Michigan Press.

Park, Shelley. 2006. "Adoptive Maternal Bodies: A Queer Paradigm for Rethinking Mothering?" *Hypatia* 21 (1): 201–26.

Parry, Diana C. 2005. "Work, Leisure, and Support Groups: An Examination of the Ways Women with Infertility Respond to Pronatalist Ideology." *Sex Roles* 53 (5-6): 337–46.

Pfeffer, Naomi. 1993. *The Stork and the Syringe: A Political History of Reproductive Medicine.* Cambridge, UK: Polity Press.

Ragone, Helena. 2000. "Of Likeness and Difference: How Race is Being Transfigured by Gestational Surrogacy." In *Ideologies of Motherhood: Race, Class, Sexuality, Nationalism,* edited by Helena Ragone and France Winddance Twine, 56–75. New York: Routledge.

Rapp, Rayna. 1988. "Moral Pioneers: Women, Men, and Fetuses on a Frontier of Reproductive Technology." *Women and Health* 13 (1-2): 101–16.

———. 1999. *Testing Women, Testing the Fetus: The Social Impact of Amniocentesis in America.* New York: Routledge.

Rich, Adrienne. 1976. *Of Woman Born: Motherhood as Experience and Institution.* New York: W. W. Norton.

Roberts, Dorothy. 1997. *Killing the Black Body: Race, Reproduction, and the Meaning of Liberty.* New York: Vintage Books.

Rothman, Barbara Katz. 2000a. *The Book of Life: A Personal and Ethical Guide to Race, Normality and Implications of the Human Genome Project.* Boston: Beacon Press.

———. 2000b. *Recreating Motherhood.* 2nd ed. New Brunswick, NJ: Rutgers University Press.

———. 2005. *Weaving a Family: Untangling Race and Adoption.* Boston: Beacon Press.

Rotstein, Gary. 1997. "Baby Boom or Baby Bust: Seeking Treatment a Matter of Cash and Culture." Part I of a Special Report on Infertility. *Pittsburgh Post-Gazette. www.post-gazette.com/babyboom.*

Ruddick, Sara. 1989. *Maternal Thinking: Toward a Politics of Peace.* Boston: Beacon.

Russo, Nancy Felipe. 1976. "The Motherhood Mandate." *Journal of Social Issues* 32 (3): 143–53.

Sandelowski, Margarete. 1991. "Compelled to Try: The Never-Enough Quality of Conceptive Technology." *Medical Anthropology Quarterly* 5 (1): 29–40.

Seidman, Steven. 2004. *Contested Knowledge: Social Theory Today.* 3rd ed. Oxford, UK: Blackwell Publishing.

Silliman, Jael, Marlene Greber Fried, Loretta Roass, and Elena R. Gutierrez. 2004. *Undivided Rights: Women of Color Organize for Reproductive Justice.* Cambridge, MA: South End Press.

Simonds, Wendy S. 2002. "Watching the Clock: Keeping Time during Pregnancy, Birth, and Postpartum Experiences." *Social Science and Medicine* 55 (4): 559–70.

Simonds, Wendy, Barbara Katz Rothman, and Bari Meltzer Norman. 2007. *Laboring On: Birth in Transition in the United States.* New York: Routledge.

Smith, Dorothy E. 1993. "The Standard North American Family: SNAF as an Ideological Code." *Journal of Family Issues* 14 (1): 50–65.

Solomon, A. 1989. "Sometimes Perganol Kills." In *Infertility: Women Speak Out about Their Experiences of Reproductive Technologies,* edited by Renate Klein, 46–50. London: Pandora Press.

Spar, Deborah. 2006. *The Baby Business: How Money, Science, and Politics Drive the Commerce of Conception.* Boston: Harvard Business School Press.

Stacey, Judith. 1996. *In the Name of the Family.* Boston: Beacon Press.

———. 2011. *Unhitched: Love, Marriage, and Family Values from West Hollywood to China.* New York: New York University Press.

Steinberg, Deborah Lynn. 1997. "A Most Selective Practice: The Eugenic Logics of IVF." *Women's Studies International Forum* 20 (1): 33–48.

Stephen, Elizabeth Hervey, and Anjani Chandra. 2000. "Use of

Infertility Services in the United States: 1995." *Family Planning Perspectives* 32 (3): 132–37.

———. 2006. "Declining Estimates of Infertility in the United States: 1982–2002." *Fertility and Sterility* 86 (3): 516–23.

Strathern, Marilyn. 1992. *Reproducing the Future: Anthropology, Kinship, and the New Reproductive Technologies.* New York: Routledge.

Szkupinski-Quiroga, Seline. 2002. "Disrupted Bodies: The Effect of Infertility on Racialized Identities." PhD diss. Dept. of Anthropology, University of California–Berkeley.

———. 2007. "Blood is Thicker than Water: Policing Donor Insemination and the Reproduction of Whiteness." *Hypatia* 22 (2): 143–61.

Tingen, Candace, Joseph B. Stanford, and David B. Dunson. 2004. "Methodologic Statistical Approaches to Studying Human Fertility and Environmental Exposure." *Environmental Health Perspectives* 112 (1): 87–93.

Thompson, Becky. 1994. *A Hunger So Wide and So Deep: African American Women Speak Out on Eating Problems.* Minneapolis: University of Minnesota Press.

Thompson, Charis. 2002. "Fertile Ground: Feminists Theorize Infertility." In *Infertility around the Globe: New Thinking on Childlessness, Gender, and Reproductive Technologies,* edited by Marcia C. Inhorn and Frank van Balen, 52–78. Berkeley: University of California Press.

———. 2005. *Making Parents: The Ontological Choreography of Reproductive Technologies.* Cambridge, MA: Massachusetts Institute of Technology.

Traver, Amy E. 2008. "Gender and International Adoption." Sociologists for Women in Society Fact Sheet. *www.socwomen.org/wp-content/uploads/2010/05/fact_fa112008-adoption.pdf.*

Turner, Bryan S. 1995. *Medical Power and Social Knowledge.* 2nd ed. London: Sage.

Twine, France Winddance. 2000. "Bearing Blackness in Britain: The Meaning of Racial Difference for White Birth Mothers of African-Descent Children." In *Ideologies of Motherhood: Race, Class, Sexuality,*

Nationalism, edited by Helena Ragone and France Winddance Twine, 76–110. New York: Routledge.

Ulrich, Miriam, and Ann Weatherall. 2000. "Motherhood and Infertility: Viewing Motherhood through the Lens of Infertility." *Feminism and Psychology* 10 (3): 323–36.

Umberson, Diane, Tetyana Pudrovska, and Corinne Reczek. 2010. "Parenthood, Childlessness, and Well-Being: A Life Course Perspective." *Journal of Marriage and Family* 72 (3): 612–29.

van Balen, Frank. 2002. "The Psychologization of Infertility." In *Infertility around the Globe: New Thinking on Childlessness, Gender, and Reproductive Technologies,* edited by Marcia C. Inhorn and Frank van Balen, 79–98. Berkeley: University of California Press.

Veevers, J. E. 1973. "Voluntarily Childless Wives: An Exploratory Study." *Sociology and Social Research* 57: 356–66.

———. 1980. *Childless by Choice.* Toronto: Butterworth.

Welter, Barbara. 1966. "The Cult of True Womanhood: 1820–1860." *American Quarterly* 18 (2): 151–74.

Yung, Judith. 1995. *Unbound Feet: A Social History of Chinese Women in San Francisco.* Berkeley, CA: University of California Press.

Zabin, Laurie Schwab, George R. Huggins, Mark Emerson, and Vanessa E. Cullins. 2000. "Partner Effects on a Woman's Intention to Conceive: 'Not With This Partner.'" *Family Planning Perspectives* 32 (1): 39–45.

INDEX

Numbers in **bold** refer to tables.